MW00844616

DR. PAUL CLAYTON

LET YOUR FOOD BE YOUR PHARMACO-NUTRITION

THE NEW ROAD TO HEALTH, HEALING AND HAPPINESS

Published by
Paul Clayton Education
Oxford

2019

"LET YOUR FOOD BE YOUR
PHARMACO-NUTRITION
The new road to health, healing and happiness."

2d edition, English UK,
Copyright © 2019 Paul Clayton Education Ltd.,
Oxford,
UNITED KINGDOM
www.drpaulclayton.eu

ISBN: 978-1-9164112-0-3
Editor: Ugnė Naujokaitytė

I was a clinical pharmacologist working with pharmaceuticals until I started to realise, in the 1970's, that the pharmacological effects of foods and food extracts are far more diverse and far more important for our health than any drug company products.

For the last 40 years, I have studied how what we eat influences our health, how the modern diet damages it, and how to put it right. This book is an overview of where the science is now. A very small part of it refers to my own work. But most of it is a summary of the work of many thousands of other scientists, working in labs and hospitals all over the world, who have been quietly assembling a new medical model.

This new model does not rely on drugs, but uses simple nutritional tools to reduce illness and support the body's ability to heal. It is more effective, more cost-effective and above all kinder than the failing system we suffer from today. And it offers hope to all of us of a better, healthier life.

Dr. Paul Clayton

Content

"Inflammation is an underlying contributor to virtually every chronic disease... rheumatoid arthritis, Crohn's disease, diabetes and depression, along with major killers such as heart disease and stroke."

Scientific American (2009)

Preface

The ancient Greek, Roman and Islamic physicians believed that our bodies contained just four different humours, or liquids, and that all illnesses were due to an imbalance between these four. This simple theory lasted some 2000 years, with traces of it lingering on until the advent of modern medicine in the 19th century. Then began a series of detailed investigations into how and what we are; which produced a hugely complex mass of information about diseases, numerous medical specialities and specialists, and the wide range of specific and generally toxic drugs which dominate today's health care system.

Unfortunately the pharmaceutical approach, although often effective in suppressing the symptoms of disease, has failed to prevent the astonishing increases in degenerative diseases that are overhelming our health care services today. Non-communicable (as opposed to infectious) diseases such as heart disease, diabetes, cancer, dementia, osteoporosis and arthritis; malfunctions of the immune system such as allergy and autoimmune disease; the neuro-developmental disorders, and mental illnesses such as depression and anxiety states (also known as 'diseases of civilization') are all spinning out of control. They are affecting more and more of us, and at earlier ages.

Current research reveals that most cases of these diseases – perhaps as many as 90% – are caused by lifestyle and dietary factors, and are largely avoidable. They have little to do with ageing per se, which is inevitable. Instead, they are largely driven by chronic, sub-clinical inflammation, a condition that is not inevitable at all. In fact, it is easy to treat, and to prevent.

This has lead to a new unifying theory of disease, a theory that leaves harmful drugs behind and focuses instead on the foods we eat. It is suprisingly simple, and could almost be compared to a modern and scientific version of the old humour theory. There are five basic elements in this new Grand Unifying Theory of disease, most of which are widely recognized.

1. The 'diseases of civilisation' are hugely influenced by lifestyle and nutritional factors.

2. Most of these diseases have a common element; chronic inflammation, a process that damages and destroys healthy tissue in every organ that it touches.

3. Three of the key anti-inflammatory compounds in our diet are the omega 3 fatty acids that occur primarily in oily fish; the polyphenols, valuable nutrients found in fruits, nuts, vegetables and spices; and the 1-3, 1-6 beta glucans found in yeasts and mushrooms.

4. The study of dietary shift (the way our diet changes over time) has revealed that levels of these anti-inflammatory nutrients have reached an all-time low. The critical ratio of omega 3 to omega 6 fatty acids in our diet has fallen by over 90%, our intake of polyphenols has declined by about the same amount, and levels of 1-3, 1-6 beta glucans in our diet have collapsed. As all three anti-inflammatory nutrients have been effectively removed from our diet, it is hardly surprising that the diseases caused by inflammation have increased. At the same time, levels of pro-inflammatory compounds in our diet have increased, due to changes in food processing.

5. When the anti-inflammatory omega 3 fatty acids, polyphenols and 1-3, 1-6 beta glucans are put back into the diet, and pro-inflammatory foods are avoided, rates of these diseases (in both animals and humans) fall by up to 90%. We become almost immune to degenerative disease, and much more resistant to infection and to allergy. When this happens, our chances of successful ageing increase dramatically.

If you want to improve your chances of living a long and healthy life, you should consider making some simple changes. Government recommendations include eating more fruit, vegetables and oily fish, cutting down on fried and grilled foods, reducing salt and alcohol, and stopping smoking. But all of this will only get you to first base. If you want to do better, and for longer, you should also take two basic anti-inflammatory supplements.

The first of these is a fish oil/ polyphenol combination, and the second is a beta glucan formulation.

I Chapter
What is inflammation?

Very few of us die of old age. The vast majority of us sicken and die prematurely, picked off by so-called 'natural causes' long before our biological life span has run its course. Cell culture studies, and the small but growing numbers of individuals who live on healthily into their second century, indicate that our potential life span may be up to 30% longer than what we consider to be normal today. But why is such a long and healthy life so rare? Why do so few of us live out our biological potential?

We used to die, in the main, of infection, starvation or trauma. Twentieth century sanitation, social progress, vaccines and to a lesser extent medicines scored significant victories against these killers – although the infectious diseases show signs of making a comeback, due to the careless way we use antibiotics and the prospect of emergent viruses. But at the time of writing, the main causes of illness and death are, still, the degenerative diseases. The pharmaceutical industry has failed to provide cures for any of these, for two principal reasons. Firstly, drugs are intrinsically unsuited to treating diseases caused not by single microbes but by multiple metabolic errors, which are in turn driven by multiple lifestyle factors. Secondly, there are no drugs available today which safely target chronic, sub-clinical inflammation. However, not **all** inflammation is bad ...

I. 1 Acute vs Chronic Inflammation

There are two fundamental kinds of inflammation, acute and chronic. Acute inflammation is generally a positive and short-lasting process, and is involved in healing and the removal of potentially harmful pathogens. Chronic inflammation is exclusively a bad thing. It involves some of the same biochemistry as the acute inflammatory reaction, but instead of healing and killing off harmful bacteria and viruses, it smoulders on for years. This causes the slow destruction of tissues in the heart, brain, cartilage, bones or elsewhere, which will eventually surface as a degenerative disease.

Accute inflammation

Acute inflammation is the rapid response of a tissue to injury. Acute inflammation can be regarded as the first line of defense against injury and is characterized by changes in the microcirculation: exudation of fluid and emigration of leukocytes (white blood cells) from blood vessels to the area of injury. Acute inflammation is typically of short duration, and it is aimed primarily at removing the injurious agent.

The five signs of acute inflammation – 'P.R.I.S.H.'

• **Pain** – the inflamed area is likely to be painful, especially when touched. Chemicals that stimulate nerve endings are released, making the area much more sensitive.

• **Redness** – this is because the capillaries fill up with more blood than usual.

• **Immobility** – there may be some loss of function.

• **Swelling** – caused by an accumulation of fluid.

• **Heat** – as with the reason for the redness, more blood in the affected area makes it feel hot to the touch.

A cut in the skin, which produces an opening to infection, causes an acute inflammatory response. Infection-fighting cells of the innate immune system congregate around the wound and release a series of biologically active compounds. Some of these increase blood flow to the area, while others cause fluid to flow in from surrounding tissues. This attracts immune cells and other factors that help to repair the wound and kill any invaders. The warm and swollen area around the cut is a sign that the immune system is working to keep the body safe, and to initiate healing.

If all goes well, and the acute imflammatory response is able to neutralize and remove the original trigger factor, inflammation stops and the healing process is completed. Some trigger factors, however, cannot be resolved – and in those who follow an unhealthy lifestyle, the trigger factors keep on coming. Now the inflammation changes, and goes 'dark'. It turns into chronic, sub-clinical inflammation. This is medical-speak for inflammation that persists, but smoulders away underground so that we are generally not aware of it until it has done so much damage that clinical symptoms finally begin to appear. These symptoms start to occur relatively late in the development of degenerative diseases, so that by the time a doctor is notified the disease has already done a good deal of damage.

Chronic inflammation

Chronic sub-clinical inflammation is an extremely complex process, but we can simplify it by describing many of the cellular structures, enzymes and messenger compounds involved in the process, as the 'inflammazone'. * In turn, the inflammazone can be divided into two functional compartments, or phases.

In the first phase, events are largely determined by the ratio of the different types of fatty acids in the membranes of your cells, which

---

* Not to be confused with the 'inflammasome', a group of small proteins that detects pathogens and other harmful elements, and triggers (eventually) the 'inflammazone'.

reflect the proportion of these fatty acids in the diet. The fatty acids in your cell membranes are broken down into pro- or anti-inflammatory messenger compounds. The omega 3 fatty acids from seafoods break down into anti-inflammatory messengers, while omega 6 fatty acids (derived from plant oils) break down into pro-inflammatory messengers. If the diet contains an excess of omega 6 fatty acids from plant oils, and not enough omega 3's, the balance of messengers is pro-inflammatory. The omega 6 breakdown products attract a range of immune cells to the affected area, and cause local oedema. This part of the process is not particularly destructive, but it activates the second phase of the inflammazone by rupturing intra-cellular structures called lysosomes. These are small vesicles filled with highly destructive enzymes called Matrix Metalloproteases (MMP's). These enzymes cause tissue damage, because when MMP's are released they erode the Extra-Cellular Matrix (ECM). It is in this second phase that the second group of anti-inflammatory dietary constituents, the polyphenols, plays such a critical role.

The ECM is a fine three-dimensional mesh of many different kinds of microfibers, including collagen and elastin, which holds all of our cells in place and in correct orientation to each other, allowing them to function in a coordinated manner and to act as a tissue or organ. This matrix is very dynamic, and is constantly being broken down and regenerated in response to the body's requirements – for example during growth or as a response to physical exercise. In chronic inflammation, however, the excessive release of MMP enzymes accelerates the rate of matrix breakdown until it outstrips the ability of the body to regenerate the matrix. Over time this leads to a slow erosion of the local matrix, and a progressive loss of functional tissue. Polyphenols have several anti-inflammatory actions here, but I will single out two of them. They inhibit the synthesis of the MMP enzymes, and they inhibit those MMP enzymes that have already been formed.

The Matrix Metallo-Proteases are the same enzymes as those released by so-called 'flesh-eating' bacteria. In someone unlucky enough to be infected by these bacteria, the sudden release of large amounts of MMP's dissolves flesh and bone, causing dramatic ulceration and loss of tissue. When small amounts of MMP's are released slowly, over decades (as occurs in chronic inflammation), they cause slow and progressive loss of tissue in bone, cartilage, the lining of artery walls, the skin – or in any other affected tissue. These tissue losses are unnoticed ('pre-clinical') to begin with, until the damage is so extensive that it starts to cause symptoms which often progress to disability and even more serious problems, such as those associated with the 'diseases of civilisation'.

As doctors are generally only called in once symptoms have become obvious, they always come late to the scene. They are like fire fighters who only ever arrive after the house has burned halfway to the ground. And once they do arrive, all they have are pharmaceutical products that treat the symptoms of disease but can never address its root causes, and come with a long and dangerous list of adverse effects. Many doctors do not yet understand that almost all the symptoms they treat have the common cause – and core – of chronic inflammation.

For example, chronic inflammation inside a joint produces slowly growing damage to the cartilage that eventually surfaces as arthritis – a medical term that simply means, inflammation inside the joint. If it occurs in bone, it will lead, over time, to osteoporosis. If in the heart and arteries, it produces atheroma and hypertension; if in the veins, vascular veins and haemorrhoids. In the bronchioles, it drives asthma, in the liver it will eventually cause hepatitis, and in the brain it will contribute to depression, and eventually surface as a neurodegenerative disease such as Alzheimer's or Parkinsons. In other words, chronic sub-clinical inflammation is the key to almost all the non-communicable diseases. The fact that it causes insidious and gradual tissue destruction is why chronic inflammation is now thought to be the main cause of almost all the age-related illnesses; and is why chronic inflammation is associated with faster ageing or „inflammageing".

The development of degenerative disease was long thought to be an intrinsic part of the ageing process; but now we can see that superficial symptoms such as the thinning of cartilage and bone, the furring of arteries and the wrinkling of skin are little to do with ageing per se. They are processes largely driven by chronic inflammation, which is driven by lifestyle and diet. Accordingly, when chronic inflammation is stopped, many of these superficial signs of ageing disappear or go into reverse as tissues start to heal. When we do this we move from the fast lane of ageing into the slow lane, where the signs of ageing are dramatically postponed and healthy middle age is extended by many years.

Look around you. You can see that some folk look a lot younger than their years, while others look much older than they really are. The fast agers not only look older, they typically have higher blood pressure, thinner bones, creakier joints, wheezier lungs – and while cosmetic surgery and Botox can reverse some of the superficial signs of ageing, their impact is merely cosmetic. The largest part of the difference between fast and slow agers is that fast ageing folk have more chronic inflammation.

Some people are at increased risk of chronic inflammation, and inflammageing. Are you:

- Over 50?

- Overweight?

- A frequent dieter?

- A smoker or a city dweller inevitably exposed to polluted air?

- A heavy consumer of baked goods, confectionary, deep-fried or fast food products?

- Have you been diagnosed with essential hypertension, or any long-term illness ending in '-itis' (which simply means inflammation)?

If you answered **yes** to any of the above, then you almost certainly have a level of chronic inflammation in your body that should be reduced <u>**now**</u> to protect your long term health.

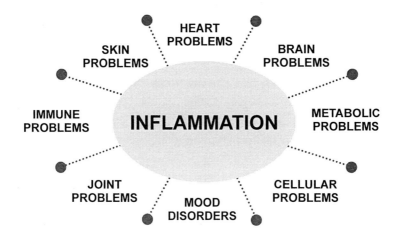

I.2 Chronic inflammation, Inflammageing and Degenerative Disease

Chronic inflammation has always been with us, but there is overwhelming evidence that as our diet has degenerated, particularly during the 20th and 21st centuries, we have become more prone to chronic inflammation and as a result, the degenerative diseases have become far more common. This is why our public health is so bad, and why the application of badly designed pharmaceuticals, administered late in the disease, has been so profoundly unsuccessful. We have partially effective, expensive (and toxic) drugs which treat the symptoms of many of our illnesses, but we have no cures – because none of today's drugs targets chronic inflammation effectively and safely. The NSAID's and corticosteroids are potent anti-inflammatory drugs but they are too toxic for preventative or long-term use. A drug that *could* suppress chronic inflammation safely would have many applications.

Chronic inflammation is so prevalent today that chronic degenerative diseases are the leading cause of mortality and morbidity throughout the world. And it is getting worse ... there is plenty of research showing that these conditions will impose an even larger burden in the future.

The largest part of this burden is caused by lifestyle and dietary factors. This has been confirmed by many studies, such as the recent Whitehall II cohort study in which researchers analysed the dietary habits of 3,775 men and 1,575 women and related this to chronic disease and mortality rates, over an average period of 16 years.

People who ate a 'Western-style' diet rich in fried and sugary foods and refined starches, aged more quickly and died younger than people who adhered to healthier diets. Ideal aging (defined as being free of chronic illness, and having high performance in physical and mental agility tests), occurred almost exclusively in the few who ate a healthier diet with plenty of fruits, vegetables, whole grains and fish. Not many consume a healthy diet, however; this healthy sub-set was a mere 4% of the total group.

Inflammageing affects all our tissues, but it is also destructive inside our cells. For example, chronic inflammation causes intoxication of the mitochondria, the power houses inside our cells that generate the energy we use to stay alive, to maintain body temperature – and to move. When mitochondria in muscle are damaged our muscles become less effective and gradually atrophy, contributing to the age-related loss of muscle known as sarcopenia. Sarcopenia contributes to metabolic ageing, and the development of metabolic syndrome and diabetes; and this in turn increases the risk of so many diseases that it cuts life expectancy by up to 8 years.

Inflammageing also shortens the telomeres, a very basic biological phenomenon that eventually prevents cells from dividing, so that tissues start to die. The powerfully anti-inflammatory omega 3's and polyphenols have both been shown to inhibit chronic inflammation, and increase telomere length.

The evidence, from many sides, is overwhelming. Reducing or preventing chronic inflammation cuts the risk of degenerative disease, and maximizes your chances of long-term health.

IMPORTANT FACTS:

• As of 2012, about half of all adults – 117 million people – had one or more chronic health conditions. One of four adults had two or more chronic health conditions.

• Seven of the top 10 causes of death in 2010 were chronic diseases. Two of these chronic diseases – heart disease and cancer – together accounted for nearly 48% of all deaths.

• Obesity is a serious health concern. During 2009–2010, more than one-third of adults, or about 78 million people, were obese (defined as body mass index [BMI] ≥30 kg/m2). Nearly one of five youths aged 2–19 years was obese (BMI ≥95th percentile).

• Arthritis is the most common cause of disability. Of the 53 million adults with a doctor diagnosis of arthritis, more than 22 million say they have trouble with their usual activities because of arthritis.

• Diabetes is the leading cause of kidney failure, lower-limb amputations other than those caused by injury, and new cases of blindness among adults.

• US citizens have the highest omega 6:3 ratios in the West, thanks to their addiction to fast foods. This explains why Americans, who are only 5% of the world's population, swallow 50% of the world's pharmaceuticals and 80% of all prescription pain-killers.

Source: https://www.cdc.gov/chronicdisease/overview/ and Mayo Clinics 2018

I.3 Is Chronic Inflammation Avoidable? History says 'Yes'.

Because of the way we live today, chronic inflammation occurs in almost all adults and in increasing numbers of teenagers. But it is easily avoidable. Medical data show that chronic inflammation is very uncommon in certain areas where people follow a traditional lifestyle. These are called Blue Zones. Campodimelle in Italy, the Mt Athos Monasteries in Greece and the Kuna Islands are all Blue Zones. These are all islands in space, but the biggest known Blue Zone is an island in time. This is the Mid-Victorian Blue Zone. If we go back to 19th century mid-Victorian England, the records show that chronic inflammation hardly existed.

Heart disease and cancer are major problems today, but the English mid-Victorians were relatively free of these conditions. Their extensive public records show that the Victorians' chances of a healthy old age were better than ours, even without the modern diagnostics, surgery and drugs that we have come to rely on.

Admittedly, the first few years after birth were hazardous, but those who reached their fifth birthday had a life expectancy similar to our own. They did not die of degenerative diseases in the main, but in childbirth, in fires, of trauma and of infections spread by crowded, insanitary living conditions and polluted water supplies.

A few Victorians did develop heart disease and cancer but the figures for these diseases were very low. They were about 90% less than they are today, in a population that lived almost as long as we do. Most of the population enjoyed relative freedom from degenerative disease, and lived healthier lives for longer than we do today. The reason? They ate a diet rich in omega 3 fatty acids, polyphenols and 1-3, 1-6 beta glucans, natural anti-inflammatory compounds that provided extensive protection against chronic inflammation. At the same time, their diet was low in the pro-inflammatory compounds that are found in so many of today's processed foods.

The evidence for this was presented in a series of scientific papers I co-wrote with the eminent historian Dr Judith Rowbotham, which were published in the Journal of the Royal Society of Medicine and the International Journal of Environmental Health and Public Health.

We were able to show that contrary to received opinion, modern medicine has not made our lives healthier. Our findings demonstrated that life expectancy today has, in some groups, fallen back from its high point in the late 19th century; and our health expectancy – the number of years we can expect to live in good health – has fallen even further.

Our Key Findings

Analysis of the mid-Victorian period in the U.K. revealed that healthy life expectancy for males at the age of 5 was roughly 3 years better than for males today (in the equivalent socioeconomic group), and their incidence of degenerative disease was roughly 10% of ours. (Women have gained 3 years, due to the development of contraception and improved gynecology). They had relatively little access to alcohol and tobacco. Their levels of physical activity and hence calorific intakes were approximately twice ours, and due to their correspondingly higher intake of fruits, whole grains, oily fish and vegetables, they consumed levels of micro- and phytonutrients at approximately ten times the levels considered normal today. This diet provided high levels of anti-inflammatory compounds, which contributed to the Victorians' freedom from degenerative disease; and provides a blueprint for nutritional and health improvement today.

The mid-Victorian period is usually defined as the years between 1850 and 1870, but in nutritional terms we identified a slightly longer period, lasting until around 1895. During these 45 years a generation grew up with probably the best standards of health ever enjoyed by a modern state.

Although the British population had risen significantly and had become increasingly urbanised, the great public health movement had not yet been established and Britain's towns and cities were still notoriously unhealthy environments. But despite this, and contrary to historical tradition, we found, using a range of historical evidence, that Britain and its world-dominating empire were supported by a workforce, an army and a navy comprised of individuals who were healthier, fitter and stronger than we are today. They were almost entirely free of the degenerative diseases which maim and kill so many of us, and although it is commonly stated that this is because they all died young, the reverse is true; public records reveal that they lived as long – or longer – than we do in the 21st century.

These findings are remarkable, as this brief period of great good health predates not only the public health movement but also the great 20th century medical advances in surgery, infection control and drugs. They are also in marked contrast to popular views about Victorian squalor and disease, views that have long obscured the realities of life and death during that 'period of equipoise'.

Our research indicates that the mid-Victorians' good health was due to their superior lifestyle and diet. This period was, nutritionally speaking, an island in time; one that was created and subsequently squandered by economic and political forces. But now that we have a better understanding of the relationship between diet, inflammation and ill health, we can recreate it.

Pro- and anti-inflammatory dietary factors.

Chronic inflammation has never before been seen on the scale that we see in the world today. This is because we not only consume far lower levels of the anti-inflammatory omega 3's, polyphenols and 1-3, 1-6 beta glucans in our diets than did our ancestors, but also we are exposed to far higher levels of pro-inflammatory compounds. This higher exposure is due to modern food processing and cooking methods; for some, the prevalence of tobacco, alcoholic spirits and environmental toxins; and for many, very low levels of physical activity.

As so many of us suffer from chronic, sub-clinical inflammation, it is no wonder that the steady accumulation of tissue damage eventually surfaces in so many of us as a major health problem – and why these problems increase in frequency as we get older. But it is little to do with ageing as such, for if we ate a profoundly anti-inflammatory diet, many of the signs of ageing would simply not appear – or would appear much later.

To reduce chronic inflammation and improve our health expectancy, all we have to do is to recreate the main elements of the mid-Victorian or Blue Zone diets; they are surprisingly similar. The data show that if you do this you can reduce your levels of inflammation quickly and effectively.

The way to staying healthy, and slowing ageing, is simple and universal. It starts with using nutritional inputs to damp the fires of inflammation, and avoiding known pro-inflammatory factors. The following chapters show how you can achieve this.

I.4. The Causes of Inflammation.
5 Key Factors

So far we have talked about chronic inflammation as the consequence of a failed acute inflammatory response. The most common causes of chronic inflammation today, however, are 5 lifestyle factors.

1. Imbalance between Omega-3 and Omega-6 fatty acids

Nutritionists call omega-6 and omega-3 fatty acids "essential" nutrients. The human body needs them for many functions, from building healthy cells to maintaining a healthy heart and brain, but we cannot produce them and must therefore obtain them from the foods we eat. The omega 6 fatty acids produce compounds which are generally pro-inflammatory, while the omega 3 fatty acids break down in the body to produce compounds which are broadly anti-inflammatory.

This is why the balance between omega 6 and omega 3 fatty acids in the diet is crucial in determining whether the environment inside our bodies is pro- or anti-inflammatory. The records indicate that for most of recorded history we consumed omega 6 and 3 fatty acids in almost equal amounts, but starting around 1900 omega 6 fatty acids in the diet increased while omega 3 fatty acids fell. The 6:3 ratio in Europe has risen from 1:1 to 15:1, and in the USA the ratio has reached an average of 25:1. Americans therefore have even more chronic inflammation than we do in Europe, and this helps to explain why US citizens, who account for a mere 5% of the global population, consume 54% of the world's pharmaceuticals, 80% of all prescription pain-killers and a disproportionate amount of anti-depressants.

The major omega-3 fatty acids are **alpha-linolenic acid** (ALA), **eicosapentaenoic** (EPA), and **docosahexaenoic acid** (DHA).

The primary source of omega-3 fatty acids in the diet is ALA, but this is not very useful as our ability to convert ALA into the important EPA and DHA is very limited when we consume excess amounts of omega 6's.

EPA and DHA are found almost exclusively in oily fish, which do not produce omega 3's but obtain them from the marine algae at the base of the cold-water marine food chain.

Omega-6 mostly comes as linoleic acid (LA) from plant oils such as corn oil, soybean oil, and sunflower oil, as well as from nuts and seeds. These oils are cheap, which is one reason why they have been poured into so many processed foods. But by driving up the 6:3 ratio in our diet to excessive levels, the manufacturers of processed foods have inflicted terrible damage on our public health.

To make matters worse, the majority of animals raised for human consumption are fed on soy and corn-based feeds. As a result, most cows, pigs and battery chickens are packed with LA and its pro-inflammatory metabolite, Arachidonic acid (AA); and their milk, meat and eggs have an unhealthily high 6 to 3 ratio. Grass-fed animals have better levels of Omega 3 but today only sheep are consistently raised this way. (Free-range chickens consume more Omega 3 fatty acids and produce meat and eggs with a better Omega 6 to 3 ratio than battery chickens.)

2. Not enough fruits and vegetables

Fruits and vegetables are important because they contain, amongst other compounds, **polyphenols.** These exert powerful anti-inflammatory effects in the body.

Polyphenols block the key enzymes that drive inflammation. These include COX-1 and COX-2, the same enzymes that are targeted by many anti-inflammatory drugs. They also block a second pair of pro-inflammatory enzymes called LIPOX-5 and LIPOX-8. Perhaps even more critically, they block a third group of pro-inflammatory and highly destructive enzymes called the matrix metallo-proteases (MMPs).

This three-way blocking action exerts a more fundamentally protective effect than any pharmaceutical drug because MMPs are directly responsible for the tissue damage that turns chronic inflammation into tissue damage which, over time, causes degenerative disease.

The Victorians ate an average of 9 to 10 portions of fruit and vegetables per day. They had large appetites, due to their high levels of physical activity. The fruits and vegetables they ate were organic, and they were heirloom varieties which contained up to three times the amounts of polyphenols of the much sweeter fruits and vegetables we eat today. We consume, on average, about 3 portions of fruit and vegetables per day. The math is simple; we have reduced consumption of these foods by about 2/3, and the polyphenol levels in what we do eat has also fallen by about 2/3. This indicates that our intake of polyphenols has fallen by around 90%.

So how much fruit and vegetables should we eat for better health? It depends on whom you talk to ...

According to one report, we should all be aiming for at least seven portions of fruit and vegetables a day. The study, carried out by researchers at University College London, analysed information from more than 65,000 adults aged 35 years or older who responded to the Health Survey for England. Researchers then followed up participants for an average of 7.7 years after their initial participation.

This study found that people who ate seven or more portions of fruit or vegetables a day had a 33% reduced risk of death from any cause, a 25% reduced risk of death from cancer and a 31% reduced risk of death from cardiovascular disease, compared with people who ate less than one portion per day (a portion is defined as 80 grams).

The American Cancer Institute goes further, and recommends nine portions of fruit and vegetables a day to reduce the risk of cancer. The Victorian data suggest that if these are heirloom varieties, that should be enough; but if you are eating modern strains, 9 portions will only get you a third of the way to the levels the Victorians consumed which, when combined with the right omega 6/3 ratio, plus significant amounts of the beta glucans, rendered them almost immune to degenerative disease.

SUMMARY

The critically important anti-inflammatory polyphenols are not present in our food in adequate amounts. Combined with the excess Omega 6 to 3 ratio in our diet and in our bodies, this creates the conditions for the perfect inflammatory storm. Add pro-inflammatory factors such as smoking and pro-inflammatory compounds found in processed and junk foods, and you are on the road to inflammageing, and accelerated ageing.

In contrast, if your diet contains enough Omega 3 to help create the right anti-inflammatory hormones, enough polyphenols to block the key inflammatory enzymes and enough 1-3, 1-6 beta glucans to maintain a healthy immune system, chronic inflammation is minimized, and natural healing processes in the body can once again predominate.

But it is not only what you eat. How you cook it is also important, as this is the way to reduce your exposure to a range of pro-inflammatory factors.

3. Pro-inflammatory cooking methods: AGE's and ALE's

When foods containing proteins are cooked at high temperatures, the protein binds with glucose or other sugars in the food to produce compounds called Advanced Glycation End products, or AGE's.

Many foods brown at high temperatures and this discolouration is a sign of AGE production. AGE compounds are very pro-inflammatory – and very ageing.

Well known AGE compounds include acrylamide, which forms when starchy foods are cooked at high temperatures and is found in crisps, French fries, toast and other foods; and PhiP, which is formed when meats are cooked at high temperatures. Both PhiP and Acrylamide have been classified as carcinogenic in humans.

AGE's can also be formed within the body when levels of glucose are too high for too long, as happens in diabetes.

In non-diabetics, enzymes bind glucose molecules to proteins, forming glycoproteins that are essential to normal body functioning. But when blood sugar levels are too high, glucose can bind to proteins in the body through non-enzymatic action. This drives the formation of AGE's and thus leads to inflammation – which explains why diabetics suffer from excessive inflammation, increased risk of serious disease and accelerated ageing.

AGE's stimulate inflammation, but this is not the only way they accelerate the ageing process. The binding of glucose to proteins causes cross-linking between proteins, binding them together in a random and dysfunctional manner. This shows up externally as skin ageing, wrinkling and reduced elasticity. Internally, it drives health problems such as cataracts, hypertension, blood clotting and kidney damage.

It is not just AGE's we have to guard against. When fats and oils are heated to high temperatures, ALE's (Advanced Lipoxidation End products) are created. These might sound friendlier but they are just as harmful and are highly pro-inflammatory. Higher levels of AGE's and ALE's in the blood are linked to higher rates of many degenerative diseases.

Foods containing high levels of both AGE's and ALE's include:

- High-temperature cooked foods rich in fats and protein: ie deep-fried, shallow-fried, broiled, seared and grilled meat, poultry and fish

- Many margarines

- French fries, chips, fried eggs (better scramble or boil them!)

- Processed foods that are mass-produced, hence cooked at speed and therefore at high temperatures. These include the spray-(=heat)-dried milk used in infant formula, and high fat spreads such as cream cheese and mayonnaise.

- smoked and cured foods

From this list you can see that most fast food staples are rich sources of AGE's and ALE's, and therefore a fast track to inflammageing. This is a good reason to cook your own food, at domestic (ie lower) temperatures. You can do even better by modifying your cooking techniques. AGE-formation is significantly reduced by cooking with moist heat, using shorter cooking times, cooking at lower temperatures, and by adding acidic ingredients such as lemon juice or vinegar.

The good news is that we don't all have to become Puritans. The aim is balance.

Humans (and other omnivores) like high-fat, high-sugar foods, and for many, life without the occasional hamburger, cake, or French fry would be rather less enjoyable. If you consciously balance those foods with anti-inflammatory foods and nutrients, you can indulge occasionally without harm.

4. Being overweight or obese

Obesity is one of the greatest public health challenges of the 21st century, and has been identified as the number two cause of premature death world-wide (after dysnutrition). It significantly increases the risk of chronic diseases such as cardiovascular disease, type-2 diabetes, hypertension, coronary heart diseases, liver and kidney disease, and a range of cancers. Its prevalence has tripled in many countries of the WHO European Region since the 1980s, and the numbers of those affected continue to rise at an alarming rate, particularly among children.

For specific individuals, obesity may further be linked to a wide range of psychological problems and stresses. For society as a whole, it has substantial direct and indirect costs that put a considerable strain on healthcare and social resources.

The challenge of obesity - quick statistics

• According to World health organization, the worldwide prevalence of obesity nearly doubled between 1980 and 2008. According to country estimates for 2008, over 50% of both men and women in the WHO European Region were overweight, and roughly 23% of women and 20% of men were obese.

• Based on the latest estimates in European Union countries, overweight affects 30-70% and obesity affects 10-30% of adults.

• Estimates of the number of overweight infants and children in the WHO European Region rose steadily from 1990 to 2008. Over 60% of children who are overweight before puberty will be overweight in early adulthood. Childhood obesity is strongly associated with risk factors for cardiovascular disease, type 2 diabetes, orthopedic problems, mental disorders, underachievement in school and lower self-esteem.

Source: http://www.euro.who.int/en/health-topics/noncommunicable-diseases
obesity/dataand-statistics)

Overweight and obesity are major causes of chronic inflammation today. This is because excess adipose tissue (fat) secretes pro-inflammatory hormones called adipocytokines. In a society where around 30% of people are obese and 62% are officially overweight, the pro-inflammatory role of fat has become an important cause of ill health and accelerated ageing. Our expanding waistlines are linked to high intakes of pro-inflammatory, processed foods high in sugars and Omega 6 fats, and to our generally low level of physical activity, which itself is pro-inflammatory.

But not all fat is the same. If you are consuming high levels of phytonutrients such as carotenoids, xanthophylls and lipophilic poplyphenols, your adipose tissue is protected and does not produce the pro-inflammatory hormones. Fat protected in this way is typically coloured yellow or orange, derived from the similarly coloured phytonutrients. Problems arise, however, in people who get fat on junk (or processed) foods. These nutrient-lite foods typically do not contain enough of the necessary phytonutrients, leaving body fat white to pearl in colour. This fat is pro-inflammatory, and dangerous.

Since most excess fat today is pro-inflammatory, and chronic inflammation is so very damaging, it is hardly surprising that being overweight is a risk factor for so many serious health problems.

The good news is that an anti-inflammatory food regime is also a weight loss regime.

5. Free Radicals

Most people have heard that free radicals can damage your health – but what are free radicals?

Free radicals are minute particles formed during the billions of chemical processes that take place in the human body, and make life possible. We are made of molecules that are in turn made up of atoms, and both molecules and atoms have electrons surrounding them. Electrons are generally paired, but during certain reactions one electron may become detached. The remaining atom (or molecule) now becomes an unstable 'free radical', with one unpaired electron. To become stable again, the free radical must grab an electron from another molecule, but now that other molecule becomes a free radical! This chain reaction of molecules stripping electrons from each other continues, sometimes reaching thousands of events long and wreaking destruction until the sequence ends.

The process of free radical formation is also called oxidative damage, as oxygen molecules are often involved. Iron rusting, fats turning rancid or a cut apple turning brown are all examples of oxidative/free radical damage.

It is only an excess of free radicals that is damaging to our health. Some level of free radical action is normal and a necessary part of the immune response to pathogens such as bacteria and viruses. Excess free radical action, on the other hand, can indeed cause cell and tissue damage, chronic inflammation and, eventually, major health problems affecting many tissues. There are a number of well-known factors that increase the levels of free radicals in our bodies, which include smoking, exposure to radiation (eg ultra-violet, X-rays and all things radioactive) – and inflammation.

When cells are damaged by inflammation they produce toxic compounds that trigger the release of excess free radicals. The resulting oxidative stress further damages those cells, and this process releases a second wave of inflammatory compounds.

This vicious circle drives both disease and the ageing process itself – unless sufficient anti-inflammatory and anti-oxidant defences are in place. This is accepted by most scientists today. Researchers at the Centre for Environmental and Health Science in Australia are very much in line with current expert opinion when they state that ageing and age-related diseases are driven by the vicious circle of chronic inflammation creating free radicals creating further inflammation.

CHRONIC INFLAMMATION ▸▸ EXCESS FREE RADICALS ▸▸ MORE INFLAMMATION

Excessive free radical load

The best-known lifestyle factor that exposes us to excessive levels of free radicals is smoking. Smoking is a leading cause of illness, accelerated ageing and death, but exposure to high levels of industrial smokes and other air pollutants can also trigger oxidative damage and chronic inflammation. For example, city dwellers exposed to high levels of diesel exhaust particulates are also at risk. Excessive exposure to ionizing radiation is another factor, which is behind government advice to be cautious with sunlight and to avoid sunburn.

Having said that, there is good evidence that much of the anti-sunlight scare is wrong. There is a long list of 'science-based' policies used by governments to try to change public behaviour, which have turned out to be counter-productive.

The advice to avoid cholesterol, for example, has been a disaster. American scientists who received funding from the sugar industry distorted their data in order to show up cholesterol and animal fats as the causes of heart disease, and to destroy the career of Professor John Yudkin, a British scientist who had accurately identified sugar as a prime cause of ill health in the 1970's. The American sugar and academic industries were better at propaganda, and while the US government's misleading advice ensured healthy sugar sales, it also lead directly to the current epidemic of obesity, diabetes, cancer, dementia and many millions of unnecessary deaths. A diet high in animal fats is not necessarily pro-inflammatory; a diet high in sugars and starches is.

The advice to avoid sunlight originated in a genuine and understandable error of judgment, rather then as a lie designed to protect industry, but has been almost as damaging. It came from clinical experience in a Northern country with a significant Celtic population. These folk have pale skins and, often, red hair, and it was found that they had a significant risk of sunburn (inflammation of the skin), and skin cancer. It was assumed that this was due to excessive sun exposure, and this snowballed into the sun avoidance policies that are so widespread today. It was only much later that scientists found that the most dangerous form of skin cancer, melanoma, was not closely related to sun exposure; that red-haired Celts are genetically more prone to skin cancer (and some other diseases); and that bad government advice had created millions of people whose vitamin D levels were so low they had become more at risk of heart disease, cancer, auto-immune diseases and other illnesses.

A diet rich in plant foods is a diet rich in carotenoids and polyphenols, both anti-inflammatory compounds. These nutrients get into the skin, and protect it against sun damage. The rural Victorians, who consumed large amounts of these protective compounds, worked long hours in the fields but hardly experienced skin cancer. Our diet of processed and junk foods is terribly depleted in these protective compounds. This leaves our skin more prone to inflammation, and many different kinds of skin damage.

Tobacco facts

• Tobacco kills up to half of its users.

• Tobacco kills around 6 million people each year. More than 5 million of those deaths are the result of direct tobacco use while more than 600,000 are the result of non-smokers being exposed to second-hand smoke.

• Second-hand smoke is the smoke that fills restaurants, offices or other enclosed spaces when people burn tobacco products.

• In 2004, children accounted for 28% of the deaths attributable to second-hand smoke.

Source: WHO, June 2016

Reducing free radical load

If you're a smoker, kicking the habit is the first thing you should do to improve your health. If you can't quit yet, switch to e-cigarettes which appear to be less harmful. A comprehensively health-protective lifestyle should also include foods and supplements with high anti-inflammatory capacity. These foods and supplements also generally have anti-oxidant capacity, which makes choosing foods and supplements easier.

We'll look at these in detail in a later section.

II Chapter: The effects of inflammation on the body

The science is still under construction, but most scientists now believe that chronic inflammation is at the core of a very large number of diseases. A large part of the ageing process as we experience it today is driven by chronic inflammation, and the major dietary and other factors that either slow or accelerate the process are well characterised.

There is overwhelming evidence that as our diet has degenerated and we have become more prone to chronic inflammation, the non-communicable diseases have become far more common.

II.1. Heart problems

Heart problems are sometimes described as 'plumbing' problems – plaque builds up in the walls of blood vessels, clogs and blocks them. But blood vessels are not like pipes; they are composed of living, reactive tissue, and are sensitive to damage and injury.

For example, they are highly sensitive to pro-inflammatory compounds such as AGE's and ALE's, the toxic substances formed when different types of foods are cooked at high temperatures, which were mentioned earlier.

These compounds can also be formed in the body; diabetics produce their own AGE's due to their high blood sugar levels and smokers produce ALE's internally because of the high oxidative stress in their bodies caused by smoking.

Whether eaten or formed in the body, these toxic compounds attack the linings of the blood vessels, causing inflammation and damage. Immune cells then target the damaged site, and migrate into the vessel wall where they attempt to resolve the damage.

The immune cells then typically die, and if there are high levels of AGE's and ALE's in the diet and in the bloodstream the increasing numbers of immune cells create a deposit of cellular debris. This causes further inflammation, further immune cell infiltration and more cell death. The cell remains gradually build up as atheroma, a toxic sludge rich in oxidised cholesterol compounds that came not from circulating cholesterol but primarily from the dead immune cells.

If there are too many pro-inflammatory compounds and not enough anti-inflammatory / anti-oxidant compounds in your diet, the rate at which atheroma is formed outstrips the body's ability to remove it.

Consequently, the atheroma builds up over time, forming plaque inside the artery walls that eventually restricts blood flow. If this happens in an artery supplying the heart, it can cause angina; if it supplies the brain, it can cause confusion or dizziness. If the plaques rupture, as they often eventually do, this can cause a heart attack or a stroke. The situation is exaccerbated by impaired micro-circulation in the capillary beds within the heart muscle, a critically important process which is also damaged by chronic inflammation.

The problem is made worse again by the fact that the same inflammation that damages micro-circulation and drives the formation of atheroma in the artery walls also causes them to constrict, so that there is a gradual rise in blood pressure. This forces the heart to work harder and it makes the arteries less elastic, creating a combination of effects that increases stresses, shock waves and damage within the arterial system.

Statins are not very effective because they attack the wrong target, namely cholesterol levels in the blood. Blood cholesterol is a very inaccurate biomarker, as fully half of all heart attacks occur in people with normal cholesterol levels.

There is a growing suspicion that the relatively minor protective effects of statins (and we will not talk about their adverse effects here) are due to the fact that some of them have a mild anti-inflammatory effect as well as a cholesterol-lowering action.

The role of undetected, chronic inflammation in heart disease may explain why 50% of heart attacks occur in patients with normal cholesterol levels. Elevated levels of inflammatory C-reactive protein (CRP), the amino acid homocysteine, glycosylated haemoglobin (HbA1c) and increasing arterial stiffness have been suggested as more important predictors of heart attacks.

IMPORTANT FACTS:

• Cardiovascular diseases (CVDs) are the **number 1** cause of death globally: more people die annually from CVDs than from any other cause.

• An estimated **17.5 million** people died from CVDs in 2012, representing 31% of all global deaths. Of these deaths, an estimated 7.4 million were due to coronary heart disease and 6.7 million were due to stroke.

• Most cardiovascular diseases **can be prevented** by addressing behavioural risk factors such as tobacco use, unhealthy diet and obesity, physical inactivity and harmful use of alcohol.

• Physical exercise, which stimulates the growth of micro-circulation in the heart muscle and exerts anti-inflammatory effects, lowers the risk of heart attacks and reduces mortality after a heart attack.

Source: WHO, September 2016

Recommended: an anti-inflammatory lifestyle and diet.

II.2 Metabolic problems

Failure of blood glucose control is a very major public health problem, and because it raises the risk of heart disease, strokes, dementia, renal and liver disease and various cancers, it cuts life expectancy by up to 8 years. It is one reason why life expectancy is beginning to fall in the USA, a trend that should be visible soon in Europe and elsewhere. It is, basically, a failure by the body to maintain levels of sugar (more accurately glucose) within physiological limits.

Levels of glucose in the blood must be maintained within a relatively narrow range; too low and we become comatose, too high and the glucose molecules initiate damaging glycation reactions. These cause chronic inflammation and damage to multiple tissues including blood vessels, nerves, the retina, the kidneys and the liver; in a complex and interlinking set of pathologies that cause oxidative damage, chronic inflammation, telomeric shortening and accelerated ageing. To make matters more complicated, rates of glucose entry into the blood fluctuate wildly, depending on the amount and nature of the carbohydrates and other macronutrients we eat. Rates of glucose removal from the blood can be just as erratic as they largely depend on how much glucose is needed as fuel by the muscles – and that depends on levels of physical activity. Glucose requirements by other tissues are more or less stable.

Under most conditions, blood glucose levels are satisfactorily controlled by a network of sensors and feedback loops. Eat more carbs than you need and insulin kicks in, lowering blood sugar by increasing glucose uptake into liver and muscle; consume fewer carbs and glucagon takes over, releasing glucose from the liver into the blood. So why are blood sugar problems so common today?

The answer is, a combination of eating too many carbohydrates, and taking too little exercise. Under these conditions more glucose enters the blood than can be removed, overwhelming all the checks and balances that formerly kept us healthy. To achieve better blood glucose control, we need to address both sides of this equation.

Exercise

Moderate exercise switches on multiple protective mechanisms...

Firstly, it exerts strong anti-inflammatory effects, because as muscle fibers contract they produce a master anti-inflammatory cytokine called IL-6. They also switch on the 'metabolic master-switch', AMP-Kinase.

When AMP-Kinase is activated it triggers increased burning of fuel in the mitochondria. This in turn leads to a lowering of LDL cholesterol in the blood and increased utilisation of the fats stored in adipose tissue – so that fat depots shrink. As excessive adipose tissue is pro-inflammatory, this is a long-term anti-inflammatory effect – but there is more.

Activated AMP-kinase restores insulin sensitivity, thus reducing or removing the pro-inflammatory effects of hyperglycaemia. It achieves this via two other inter-related mechanisms, both of which enhance the ability of muscle to soak up glucose from the blood stream. AMP-kinase increases the numbers of GLUT4 glucose uptake pumps on muscle cell membranes that 'pull' glucose into the muscle; and it triggers autophagy, a process of tissue renewal in the muscle that increases numbers of the mitochondria where that glucose will be 'burned'. Mitochondria are highly dynamic organelles that fuse and divide in response to environmental stimuli, developmental status, and energy requirements. The increase in mitochondria triggered by activated AMP-K explains why, when you take exercise you get fitter and achieve better blood glucose control. As blood glucose levels come under control, insulin levels fall also; and this is another anti-cancer mechanism.

Sitting down switches AMP-K off, with al the attendant ill effects. This is why sitting has been dubbed the new smoking.

Carbs

Some interesting research papers show that contrary to the diabetes associations, which are mainly funded by drug companies and may have deeply conflicting loyalties, an effective way of improving blood sugar control is to reduce the intake of sugars and refined carbohydrates. A low-glycemic diet has also been shown to reduce the risk of late complications such damage to the eye. A low-glycemic diet lowers the body's production of insulin, and insulin is, among other things, an ageing hormone. A low-carb, low-insulin lifestyle should therefore have other anti-ageing benefits, and recent research has indeed revealed that the low-glycemic diet protects against a very wide range of ageing problems. Increased exercise levels confer similar benefits.

Let me just recap the basic causes of poor blood sugar control. The typical Western diet pours excessive amounts of glucose into the bloodstream which, when combined with under-exercised muscle, together with a diet depleted in second messenger co-factors such as chromium and manganese, pretty much guarantees insulin resistance. As this diet / low exercise combination generally leads to an accumulation of adipose tissue which has an excessive omega 6:3 ratio and is unprotected by fat-soluble nutrients, that adipose tissue becomes an important source of inflammation. Growing inflammation makes the insulin resistance worse and this – together with glycation reactions – leads to accelerated ageing and a spectrum of metabolic complications which affect almost every organ and tissue in the body. A vicious cycle develops because the process of chronic inflammation and increased insulin resistance causes muscle wasting, and this makes insulin resistance worse.

Given our pathological lifestyles it is not surprising that rates of poor blood sugar control are soaring – in fact, it is surprising that they are not more prevalent. But people with this problem have a choice. They can reverse this mess of metabolic imbalances with simple lifestyle changes, with a good chance of curing themselves.

Or they can opt for a pharma approach, and suppress some of their symptoms with variously toxic drugs. The pharma approach is widely and uncritically promoted, but it is a feeble-minded and in the end a relatively ineffective strategy.

Recommendations

Take more exercise

If you crave starchy foods switch from digestible to fermentable carbs. This mostly means switching from grains and potatoes to pulses and legumes, but there are other techniques you can use. For example, by cooking, cooling and re-heating starchy foods such as potatoes, you convert the starch from digestible to fermentable. In this state it no longer converts to blood glucose, and instead develops healthy prebiotic properties. Prebiotics help to normalise the microbiome in a way which exerts primary anti-inflammatory effects in the gastro-intestinal tract and secondary anti-inflammatory effects elsewhere in the body.

IMPORTANT FACTS:

• The number of people with diabetes has risen from 108 million in 1980 to 422 million in 2014.

• The global prevalence of diabetes among adults over 18 years of age has risen from 4.7% in 1980 to 8.5% in 2014.

• Diabetes is a major cause of blindness, kidney failure, heart attacks, stroke and lower limb amputation.

• In 2012, an estimated 1.5 million deaths were directly caused by diabetes and another 2.2 million deaths were attributable to high blood glucose.

• WHO projects that diabetes will be the 7th leading cause of death in 2030.

• Healthy diet, regular physical activity, maintaining a normal body weight and avoiding tobacco use are ways to prevent or delay the onset of type 2 diabetes.

Source: WHO, November 2016

Recommended: Regular physical exercise, minimal sugars and starches, an anti-inflammatory lifestyle and diet.

II.3 Cellular problems

There is a good deal of evidence that chronic inflammation predisposes an individual to cellular problems. This review describes some of the underlying causes of the association between chronic inflammation and cancer: http://www.cancernetwork.com/review-article/chronic-inflammation-and-cancer

Here's what Scientific American said in a key article in 2008. 'Cancer begins with a series of genetic changes that prompt a group of cells to over-replicate and then invade surrounding tissue, the point at which true malignancy begins. Eventually some tumour cells may break off and establish new growths (metastases) at distant sites.'

What appears to enable that progression from DNA damage to the eventual health problem is chronic inflammation, which then encourages free radical damage. As the magazine then puts it: 'Genetic damage is the match that lights the fire, and inflammation is the fuel that feeds it'. Chronic inflammation makes a further contribution by fuelling the processes of tumor growth and spread.

Modern diets and lifestyles, which ensure that most of us have chronic inflammation, have also ensured that cancer has become the second leading cause of death world-wide (after heart disease, also driven by chronic inflammation). So what might we expect if we were to reduce our burden of chronic inflammation, and follow an anti-inflammtory regime?

To begin with, we could expect to see a substantial reduction in the risk of premature death, from all causes. Studies such as HALE showed that in subjects following a Mediterranean diet (which is anti-inflammatory), the risk of death from all causes was reduced by 66% over a ten-year follow-up.

Other data sources suggest that an even more anti-inflammatory lifestyle confers an even greater measure of protection. The mid-Victorians, who consumed far higher levels of omega 3 fatty acids and polyphenols and 1-3, 1-6 beta glucans and fiber than we do, enjoyed a very anti-inflammatory lifestyle. They ate no processed food, did not use high temperature cooking methods, did not use tobacco or alcohol nearly as much as we do, took far more exercise and did not experience obesity or even much overweight. As a result, they are reported to have had cancer levels approximately 90% lower than those we see today. This helps to explain why Victorian men lived three years longer on average than their socio-economic equivalents do today!

As both angiogenesis (essential for tumor growth) and metastatic spread involve processes that are basically inflammatory, it is easy to see how such an anti-inflammatory lifestyle afforded the Victorians such good defences against cancer – and against degenerative disease in general.

This is not the whole story. They also ate large quantities of water cress, cabbage, Brussels sprouts, onions and related vegetables that contain sulphur compounds which increase Phase 2 enzymes in the liver. This enabled the Victorians to excrete carcinogens more effectively than we do. They consumed far greater amounts than we do of a range of phytonutrients which have the ability to stop the growth of cancer cells, force them to return to normal or commit 'suicide'. As mentioned above, they smoked and drank less than we do, took more exercise, and experienced very little obesity. They were thus protected against cancer in many ways, where we are not.

IMPORTANT FACTS:

• Cancer is the second leading cause of death globally, and was responsible for 8.8 million deaths in 2015.

• The number of new cases is expected to rise by at least 70% over the next 2 decades.

• Around one third of deaths from cancer are due to 5 behavioral and dietary risks: high body mass index, low fruit and vegetable intake, lack of physical activity, tobacco and alcohol.

• Tobacco use is the most important risk factor for cancer and is responsible for approximately 22% of cancer deaths.

• The economic impact of cancer is significant and is increasing. The total annual economic cost of cancer in 2010 was estimated at approximately US$ 1.16 trillion.

• Obesity increases the risk of many cancers including cancer of the mouth, throat, esophagus, stomach, pancreas, gall bladder, kidney, womb and breast (in post-menopausal women), and the colon and rectum.

• Cancers in teens and young adults have doubled since 1950; bowel cancer has increased up to 4 times. Researchers calculate that adults born circa 1990 have double the risk of colon cancer and quadruple the risk of rectal cancer compared with those born circa 1950. By 2030, the incidence of colorectal cancer in people under 50 is expected to nearly double.

Source: WHO, February 2017

Recommended: Regular physical exercise, smoking cessation, moderate alcohol consumption, weight control, an anti-inflammatory lifestyle and diet.

II.4 Brain problems

Chronic inflammation is a significant factor in memory loss, confusion, disorientation and decline of other cognitive abilities. It is also implicated in Alzheimer's, Parkinson's and the motor neurone diseases. It was long ago suspected that the risk of these conditions was reduced in people who, because they had an inflammatory condition such as arthritis, took the anti-inflammatory drug indomethacin. Ibuprofen may also have some protective effect. These drugs are too toxic for long-term preventive use, and the evidence of their effectiveness is disputed. A diet rich in anti-flammatory nutrient, however, most certainly reduces the risk of developing serious brain problems.

Recently, for example, an extended piece of research called the Honolulu-Asia Aging Study found that men with the highest levels of inflammation, as measured by CRP, were three times more likely to develop dementia than those with the lowest levels.

The incidence of neurodegenerative diseases such as Alzheimer's, Parkinson's and motor neurone disease are rising rapidly, and the age of onset is falling. How the neurodegenerative conditions develop is the focus of intense study, and is a very complex process – there are probably three or even 4 sub-types of Alzheimer's disease alone. But we do know that chronic inflammation is involved in all of these, and that this process attacks and kills brain cells. This is supported by work at the Buck Institute in California, which shows that at patients with some sub-types of Alzheimer's respond very positively to anti-inflammatory nutrient regimes.

Inflammation in the brain is also a central part of the entire ageing process. Inflammation in a specific part of the brain called the hypothalamus seems to be particularly critical, as the hypothalamus secretes hormones that affect almost every system in the body. Inflammatory damage to the hypothalamus affects levels of these hormones including growth hormone, which controls rates of tissue growth and repair, and gonadotropin-releasing hormone (GnRH). Unsurprisingly, a fall in these hormones accelerates the ageing process;

in experimental mice, hypothalamic inflammation lead to a rapid loss of muscle strength and size, skin thickness, ability to learn – and life expectancy. Conversely, blocking inflammation in the hypothalamus slowed ageing and increased longevity by about 20%; and adding extra GnRH increased the ability of the mice to grow new brain cells.

Preventing inflammation and nerve cell damage and death in the hypothalamus is a very important anti-ageing strategy – but you don't need to treat yourself with GnRH. A number of the anti-inflammatory polyphenols have already been shown to slow or prevent brain ageing; as have the omega 3 fatty acids. It is a sure bet that the combination of omega 3 fatty acids and polyphenols will be far more effective than either nutrient on its own. In support of this, studies carried out at McMaster University in Ontario have shown that mice fed on a very nutrient-dense and anti-inflammatory diet do not experience brain ageing at all.

Dietary enhancement and exercise are particularly important because there is good evidence that obesity (which is pro-inflammatory) accelerates inflammation in the hypothalamus, which in turn causes and exacerbates diabetes. Diabetes causes further chronic inflammation, creating a further twist in a vicious circle which drives the ageing process even faster and further increases the risk of dementia. This is yet another example of how our defective diets and lifestyles create a perfect metabolic storm which drives so many of us to premature and unnecessary disability and death.

IMPORTANT FACTS:

Worldwide, **nearly 44 million** people have Alzheimer's or a related dementia. (Alzheimer's Disease International)

• Only 1 in 4 people with Alzheimer's disease have been diagnosed. (Alzheimer's Disease International)

• Neurodegenerative deaths in the over 65's increased three-fold in men, and 5-fold in women, since 1989. (Pritchard and Rosenorn-Lanng '17)

• The average age of onset of dementia has fallen by 10 years since 1995 (Pritchard and Rosenorn-Lanng '17); and is now regularly diagnosed in people as young as the late 40's.

• Alzheimer's and other dementias are the **top cause for disabilities** in later life. (Alzheimer's Disease International)

• There are over **9.9 million new cases of dementia each year worldwide**.

Source: Alzheimer's Association

Recommended: an anti-inflammatory lifestyle and diet.

II.5 Mood disorders

Depression is the number 1 illness worldwide. With 322 million cases diagnosed (and the real figures probably at least 3 times that, ie 1000 million plus), and an increase of around 20% in the last decade alone, this is a major problem and the bane of many lives. Add in stress and anxiety, which have become almost universal, and you can see that we have created an unhappy and dysfunctional society.

There are plenty of external issues that make us unhappy and anxious. Isolation, illness, difficult partners, bad bosses, corrupt and lying politicians – the list is a long one. But these have always been around, so what has changed to make depression and anxiety so universal? Changes in our diet, which have made us more prone to chronic inflammation in general, have also made us more likely to develop inflammation in the brain. And inflammation in the body and specifically in the brain has been strongly linked to both depression and anxiety.

A large-scale Danish study published in *JAMA Psychiatry* strengthens the hypothesis that mood disorders like depression are directly tied to inflammation. Researchers found that patients with an autoimmune disease (which cause chronic inflammation) were 45 percent more likely to have a mood disorder, while any history of infection increased the risk of a mood disorder by 62 percent. And about one-third of people diagnosed with a mood disorder had been hospitalized in the past for a serious infection, a condition which also causes chronic inflammation.

The most effective anti-inflammatory agents are the fish oils and the polyphenols, which work most effectively when combined – as they are in oily fish. Work by many good scientists has shown, repeatedly, that in countries where more fish is consumed, almost all types of mental illness and crimes of violence are significantly less frequent than occur in countries where fish intake is low. A very different but complementary line of evidence comes from the work on saffron, a culinary herb which reduces inflammation in specific parts of the brain and exerts powerful anti-depressant and anxiolytic effects. These benefits were first recognized 1000 years ago by the great Persian polymath Ibn Sina, known in the West as Avicenna. More recently a group of scientists in Iran (modern-day Persia) tested Avicenna's ideas and found that saffron was as powerful as Prozac, but without any safety issues. Subsequent work showed that a standardized extract of saffron (Affron) was equally effective in curing low mood states, in both adults and children; and astoundingly, was effective within 2 hours of taking the first tablet. (This extreme rapidity is because saffron works via a different and more direct route than any of the antidepressant drugs). There are 16 clinical trials to date, all confirming saffron's efficacy and safety.

Recommended: Affron, an anti-inflammatory lifestyle and diet.

II.6 Joint problems

There are around 200 types of musculoskeletal conditions, divided into seven main groups. All of these involve some degree of chronic inflammation which can affect part of or the entire joint assembly. Most of them will cause increasing damage to the affected joints over time, despite medical treatment, and may eventually require replacement surgery.

Numbers of hip and knee replacement surgeries are increasing rapidly, due to a combination of increasing obesity (which overloads the joints), and nutritional changes which have degraded cartilage metabolism and therefore quality.

The process of chronic inflammation affecting joints is, from a biochemical and cellular perspective, the same as that which might affect the heart and blood vessels, or any other tissue. Unsurprisingly, it responds to the same anti-inflammatory nutrients, specifically omega 3's and polyphenols.

Although there are no specific nutrition guidelines for people with RA, researchers have found a diet rich in omega-3 fatty acids, antioxidants and phytochemicals supplies the body with powerful anti-inflammatory nutrients. These foods are commonly part of a Mediterranean-style diet of fish, olive oil, fruits, vegetables, nuts/seeds and beans. This diet has been analyzed in small studies for its impact on joint symptoms. Results showed improvements in pain, morning stiffness, disease activity and physical function.

Cold-water fish high in omega-3s have shown to be particularly beneficial, as has olive oil. Researchers have found that polyphenols in extra virgin olive oil have a significant impact on inflammation, and reduce joint cartilage damage. Earlier studies showed that olive polyphenols inhibits the pro-inflammatory COX-1 and COX-2 enzymes, and more recently they were also shown to inhibit the tissue-destroying MMP enzymes.

IMPORTANT FACTS:

Prevalence of Arthritis

• From 2013- 2015, an estimated 54.4 million US adults (22.7%) per year were diagnosed with some form of arthritis or other inflammatory condition affecting the joints.

• The most common form of arthritis is osteoarthritis. Other common arthritic conditions include gout, fibromyalgia, and rheumatoid arthritis.

Projected Prevalence

• By 2040, an estimated 78 million (26%) US adults ages 18 years or older are projected to have doctor-diagnosed arthritis.

Leading Cause of Disability

• Arthritis and related conditions have been the most common cause of disability among US adults for the past 15 years.

Source: https://www.cdc.gov/arthritis/data_statistics/arthritis-related-stats.htm

Recommended: an anti-inflammatory lifestyle and diet.

II.7 Immune problems

Autoimmune problems are increasing at a rate of between 3 and 5% every year. There is no general agreement as to the causes of this increase; some believe that governmental advice to shun sunlight, which has contributed to widespread vitamin D depletion, may be part of the problem, while others focus on the use of micro-particulate titanium dioxide as a coloring agent in foods, cosmetics and pharmaceuticals. In any case, when the immune system attacks the body, the resulting tissue damage is driven by chronic inflammation. By switching from a pro-inflammatory to a sufficiently anti-inflammatory lifestyle and diet, it should be possible to damp the inflammatory process enough to make the immune system change course. As a former confirmed sufferer from Graves' Disease, this is something that I have personally witnessed and experienced.

Allergies have shown an even greater increase in the last two generations, doubling every decade for the last 30 years at least. The reasons for this increase are summed up by the modified hygiene hypothesis.

Even before the evolution of higher life forms, yeasts and moulds were present. Yeasts have been ever-present in the air we breathe, and on all foodstuffs we consume. This is why all higher life forms, from insects to fish to mammals, have one or more receptors on their immune cells which recognise the presence of yeast, and allow the host to defend against invasion by that yeast. Over the aeons, animal's immune systems evolved to become dependent on the presence of yeast to function effectively, and the 1-3, 1-6 beta glucans in yeast cell walls are the most potent of all immuo-modulators[1]. This applies to humans too. We have always consumed significant amounts of the 1-3, 1-6 beta glucans in fermented foods such as bread and alcoholic beverages, and lower levels of these compounds as contaminants on all other foods.

---

[1] (These are related to, but distinct from the 1-3, 1-4 beta glucans found in cereals such as oats. These have positive effects on the bacterial population in our intestines (the microbiome), but have little direct immune function.)

Cut to 1950. The post-war period brought many changes. The first synthetic fungicides were developed and by degrees, agricultural systems became chemical war zones where fungal (and yeast) contamination was effectively obliterated. Microfiltration was introduced into brewing, and the beta glucans disappeared from beers and wines. And due to our low energy lifestyles, our intakes of fermented foods such as bread, declined also.

When the 1-3, 1-6 beta glucans are removed from our diet, the adaptive immune system becomes imbalanced, and it moves from TH1 dominance to TH2 dominance. This means that the immune system becomes much more prone to react to harmless stimuli such as grass pollen. And as there has been a parallel shift from an anti- to a pro-inflammatory diet, reactions to these normally harmless stimuli have become more severe.

In the pharmaceutical magazines you sometimes see illustrations of the old jug inhalers, used to treat asthmatics in the 19th century. These illustrations are meant to show us how ridiculous old-time medicine used to be, and how sophisticated the pharmaceutical industry has become. The historical records show us, however, that back in the 19th century asthma was not only rare but it was also mild; and the steam inhalers were usually enough to get the asthma sufferer back to work (or to class) in a few minutes. There was asthma back then but it was rare because the food chain contained significant amounts of 1-3, 1-6 beta glucans, so that the immune system did not have a high tendency to malfunction. And it was mild, because our ancestors ate, until very recently, a profoundly anti-inflammatory diet.

More recent studies have shown that 1-3, 1-6 beta glucan supplements are effective in reducing the frequency and severity of symptoms. In my experience, combining this approach with an anti-inflammatory diet or supplement works even more effectively. (Certain parasitic worms have a similar effect in modulating the Th1 and Th2 cells, but most people unaccountably prefer taking a yeast supplement to swallowing parasites).

Pro tip: If you wish to consume yeast, kill it (ie microwave it) before you ingest it or you will turn into a brewery. This is less fun than it sounds. And as many people are allergic to the mannoproteins in yeast cell walls, I generally recommend a standardised and purified beta glucan extract.

Recommended: an anti-inflammatory lifestyle and an anti-inflammatory and immuno-modulating diet.

II.8 Gut problems

Gastro-intestinal problems are at an all-time high.

Constipation severe enough to require laxatives now affects more than 10% of the population, rising to almost 20% in the USA.

Then there is irritable bowel syndrome, or IBS. IBS is not a single disease but a collection of symptoms, including diarrhoea and constipation, and can be caused by stress, antibiotic use or a low-fibre, processed food diet.

Good data are hard to obtain, but it looks as if here too there has been a substantial increase since the 1950's. The global incidence is now reckoned to be between 12 and 15%; with the higher figures in developed countries where more ultra-processed foods are consumed.

Stress, antibiotic use and a low-fibre diet all affect the microbial population in the large bowel, causing it to grow excessive numbers of gram-negative bacteria. Gram-negative bacteria are not all harmful, and some of them may contribute to our health; but they are gram-negative because they are coated with lipopolysaccharides, compounds which are highly pro-inflammatory.

When the bacterial population in the large bowel becomes unbalanced, pro-inflammatory, and starts to cause symptoms, this is termed 'dysbiosis'.

This is not the only kind of dysbiosis. For example, some cases of IBS can be helped with a FODMAP[1] diet. In these cases, the IBS is probably not caused by having the wrong population of microbes in the large bowel, but by having normally healthy (gram-positive) bacteria in the wrong place, in the small bowel.

In most cases of IBS, however, there is evidence of chronic inflammation in the intestines. This is what one would expect to see if the microbial

---

[1] The FODMAP diet is a diet low in Fermentable Oligosaccharides, Disaccharides, Monosaccharides and Polyols.

balance had been damaged, and now contained excessive amounts of gram-negative bacteria.

Inflammatory bowel disease (IBD) is altogether more serious. The two major types of IBD, ulcerative colitis and Chrohn's Disease, are autoimmune diseases. They present with a good deal of chronic inflammation, combined with dysbiosis. IBD's are very different from IBS but they too are increasing, and have trebled since the 1980's.

The most serious disease of the bowel is bowel cancer, and here we see the same worrying trend; compared to those were born in the 1950's, people born in the 90's (ie the subsequent generation) have double the risk of colon cancer and four times the risk of rectal cancer. As with all the other gastrointestinal disorders listed above, these cancers are very much linked with dysbiosis and chronic inflammation.

Dysbiosis and chronic inflammation in the gut appear to be significant causes of a number of disease states. From this perspective, a nutritional strategy that restores microbial balance and is also anti-inflammatory, makes good sense.

Prior to the 20th century processed foods were not available, other than the most simple stuffs such as bread, cheese, yoghurt etc. People ate a diet that contained far more prebiotic fibres than we eat today. These fibres play a critically important role in maintaining good microbial and gut health.

Prebiotic fibres are carbohydrates, but unlike more familiar carbohydrates such as sugar and starch they cannot be digested, and are not broken down in the small intestine to form glucose. Instead, they pass intact into the large bowel where they are used as food or fuel by gram-positive bacteria such as lactobacilli, bifidobacteria and streptococcus thermophilus. If these bacteria sound familiar it is because we use them to make yoghurt and other fermented foods. They are called probiotics, although the bean-counters at the regulatory agencies don't like this term.

The probiotic gram-positive bacteria utilise the prebiotic fibres as fuel, multiply and displace and kill off gram-negative bacteria. Killing off the gram-negative bacteria reduces the amount of lipopolysaccharide in the gut, which reduces inflammation. But the prebiotic fibres have a complementary action that is just as important. When probiotic bacteria consume the prebiotic fibres, they break them down to butyric acid. Butyric acid is not only powerfully anti-inflammatory, it is very good indeed at killing cancer cells.

In this way, when prebiotic fibres switch the balance of the bacteria in the gut from gram-negative towards gram-positive, they provide anti-inflammatory and anti-cancer benefits.

This improves the situation inside the gut, and it also generates health benefits elsewhere in the body. Too much inflammation in the gut makes it 'leaky', allowing bacterial and other toxins to enter the blood stream and cause problems in other tissues. Dysbiosis has been linked to depression, autism, schizophrenia, reduced stamina, impaired blood glucose control, weight gain and Parkinson's Disease. Other problems will surely emerge.

It seems very logical to consider an anti-inflammatory approach to gut health, and the strategy is a simple one. Put prebiotic fibres back into the diet, where they always used to be, and restore a more gram-positive and less inflammatory population of bacteria in the gut.

There are many different prebiotic fibres. The best documented include FOS, inulin, 1-3, 1-4 beta glucans and resistant starch. It is always best to use a blend of these, of graded lengths and complexity. This is because shorter fibres ferment faster, while longer and more complex fibres ferment more slowly. This is important, because a carefully judged blend of fast and slow fibres will help to re-balance the bacterial population throughout the length of the large bowel.

This approach is linked to a reduced risk of almost all bowel problems. If this is not enough to persuade you, this strategy also leads to better regularity and health benefits through the body.

CAUTION: Some individuals are very sensitive to prebiotic fibres. In certain circumstances, probiotic species invade the upper (small) bowel, where they do not normally live in significant numbers. When this happens, prebiotics cause probiotic growth in the small bowel, which can be very uncomfortable. If you have this problem, you could try flushing the probiotics back into the large bowel with carrot soup, an old German remedy for stomach upsets. Boil the carrots until a slight sweetness develops. This is due to carrot carbohydrates being broken down to smaller sugar-like molecules. These appear to act as anti-adhesins; that is, they dislodge bacteria from their binding sites on the gut wall, much like cranberry juice flushes bacteria from the bladder. In my limited experience, a bowl of this soup every day for a week is sufficient. After that you should be able to switch to the prebiotic blend.

II.9 Down in the Mouth

One of the most common inflammatory conditions is gingivitis. This is the medical term for chronic inflammation of the gums. That spot of blood when you spit into the sink after cleaning your teeth is a giveaway, and so is bad breath; it's not you, it's the bacteria living around the roots of your teeth, combined (if you don't brush and floss just right) with particles of decaying food.

You shouldn't ignore that blood spot, because untreated gingivitis progresses to periodontal disease, where the bone of the jaw around the tooth or teeth is eroded. This is, so far, irreversible, and it causes more lost teeth than caries do. It also spoils your jaw line.

Almost everyone has at least a slight degree of gingivitis.

Even if your oral hygiene is good, gingivitis can still be caused by bacteria which live in the plaque and tartar that builds up around the teeth over time. This is the most common cause of gingivitis, which is why plaque control is so important. Other causes of gingivitis include medications such as phenytoin and cyclosporine, and plain old malnutrition – which is now, thanks to our low energy lifestyles and low nutrient processed foods, very common indeed. This helps to explain why almost half of all adults in the USA have periodontal disease, as they do in other countries that consume excessive amounts of processed and ultra-processed foods.

Lost teeth are bad enough, but it gets worse. Chronic inflammation in the gums produces inflammatory hormone-like compounds that leach into the saliva and these, plus a cocktail of bacterial toxins, are then swallowed. Then they pass into the bloodstream. And then, they appear to be linked to an increased risk of diabetes, heart disease, and cancers of the oesophagus, breast, pancreas and gall bladder. The risks go up even more if you combine poor oral hygiene with smoking.

A few blood spots in the sink are not the end of the world, but if the problem persists and worsens, the above health conditions become more likely.

Brushing and flossing (or using inter-dental toothbrushes), is a good investment in your long-term health. But even the best brushing technique, and even electronic toothbrushes, do not remove all plaque. And they cannot remove tartar at all. Which is why we come back to plaque. What is it? And what is tartar?

Dental plaque is a slime, or biofilm, produced by bacteria living in the mouth. These bacteria cannot be removed by brushing or by mouthwashes; the bacteria remain, because they bind fast to compounds on the surface of your gums and teeth, and in the biofilm. The biofilm acts as a bio-glue, enabling the bacteria to stay in the mouth and not be swallowed into the acid bath of your stomach - which would kill them.

Plaque itself is not so bad, and you remove most plaque on a daily basis when you brush. However, if it is allowed to remain for more than a day or so, minerals from the saliva bind to the biofilm and it calcifies, becoming tartar. This is much tougher than biofilm, and cannot be removed by brushing. So every few months you go to the dentist and have the tartar removed. This can be somewhat painful, but you do it (I hope) because you don't want more serious problems to emerge, and you want to hold on to your ivory.

Seaweed is a less painful and usually cheaper alternative. And, you can do it yourself.

Common seaweeds such as Fucus vesiculosus (bladder wrack) and wakame (used to wrap sushi) contain compounds called fucoidans that inhibit the growth of dental bacteria, and block their ability to produce biofilm. By preventing biofilm formation, the fucoidans prevent tartar build-up and protect against gingivitis. These seaweed compounds are polysulphated oligomeric carbohydrates, a factoid which you can now forget. (For the geeks, they resemble heparin and can, if consumed in very large amounts, interfere with blood clotting).

When you eat the right seaweeds, some of the fucoidans are absorbed in the gut and enter the blood stream. They then pass into the intracrevicular glands located between your teeth, and finally into the intracrevicular fluids which wash the roots of the teeth. This mechanism is part of your innate immune system, along with the acid in your stomach and the ciliated cells which line your airways. When fucoidans pass around the roots of the teeth they effectively wash them with bio-teflon, dislodging the plaque-causing bacteria and washing them away. This is similar to using cranberry juice or l-mannose to flush the urinary tract.

The fucoidans have been shown to reduce plaque and tartar in animals and in humans. They act as a sort of additional toothbrush, but they can refresh the parts ordinary toothbrushes cannot reach. And they do more. I have personally found that if taken regularly, existing tartar on the teeth simply falls off. The mechanisms are understood, and involve a kind of sabotage of the tartar-building process.

There is a final bonus. As the fucoidans circulate in the blood, they make it difficult for any bacteria that might get in there to adhere to an artificial heart valve, hip or knee joint. In this way, I am pretty certain that they reduce the risk of late post-operative sepsis.

Caution. If taken in large doses, the fucoidans can cause side effects such as extended blood clotting times. This is generally positive for most people (if you eat too much processed foods your blood clotting time is probably too short), but it is a potential problem in anyone taking blood thinners. Talk to your doctor.

Other side effects include enhanced responses to chemotherapy, and protection against the adverse effects caused by chemotherapy. These side effects are entirely positive, as you often see with natural compounds. However, should you be unlucky enough to acquire cancer and do not inform your oncologist you are taking fucoidans, you may get into trouble because many oncologists will increase the dose of therapy until it hurts. If you don't show enough signs of damage they may increase the dose and thus harm you. I've seen too many cases like this.

The fucoidans have a range of anti-cancer properties themselves, and this may explain – at least in part – why rates of some cancers are lower in countries where the brown seaweeds are commonly consumed.

II.10 Fertility - infertility

Increasing numbers of couples who want to have children are finding it harder to do so. The World Health Authority estimates that infertility affects up to 80 million couples worldwide. The problem is not universal; in some countries the trends are clearly negative while in others there has been relatively little change. The West seems to be particularly badly affected, and India (for example) has suffered a similar decline. Africa on the other hand has not yet been seen this trend; and these regional changes in fertility are one reason why some ignorant and irresponsible politicians have encouraged illegal mass migration.

One cause of falling rates of childbirth is that fertility peaks in both sexes at around 30, and more couples in the developed nations are starting families much later in life. But infertility has been increasing in younger women and men too. Female fertility has fallen in the last few years, and male testosterone levels, sperm counts and sperm quality have been falling for at least a generation. Sperm quality is a complex and composite measure, but to give a better idea of what is happening, the % of normally shaped and normally motile sperm have both declined very significantly, even in younger and 'healthy' males.

Decreasing male and female fertility (the reduced ability to make healthy sperm and eggs) are both driven by the same inter-connected set of problems; dysnutrition, obesity, changing levels of sex hormones, insulin resistance and chronic inflammation. And all of these are caused by excessively sedentary lifestyles, combined with junk food diets. In particular, the rising tide of ultra-processed food – encouraged by a criminally irresponsible food industry – has made dysnutrition, obesity and chronic inflammation almost universal. You can see the epidemic of chronic inflammation in our terrible public health statistics, and the prevalence of the degenerative diseases today. Increasing infertility is another symptom of the same problem.

Egg and sperm formation are highly complex processes, and involve carefully controlled (physiological) levels of inflammation. In contrast, excessive inflammatory and oxidative stress damages both sperm and egg formation, making it more difficult to conceive.

Certain nutrients seem to play a key role. High omega 6:3 ratios in men correlate with infertility and conversely, higher intakes of the anti-inflammatory omega 3's have been shown to improve sperm counts in men, and fertility in both men and women. Other nutrients play a role too.

Researchers from the Harvard T.H. Chan School of Public Health and Harvard Medical School recently published a review of studies that examined the impact of diet on fertility. They found that for women trying to become pregnant naturally folic acid, B12, the omega 3's and nutrient-dense, anti-inflammatory diets were linked to positive effects on fertility; while ultra-processed (and pro-inflammatory) foods had negative effects.

All in all, the evidence is quite persuasive. For couples who want to conceive, changing from an pro-inflammatory to an anti-inflammatory and nutrient-dense diet will in many cases be a better and cheaper option than resorting to medical infertility treatments.

This means cutting out junk foods, eating more unprocessed foods and taking anti-inflammatory supplements where necessary.

II.11 Children and inflammation

The same lifestyle that condemns so many of us to chronic inflammation, and thus to early onset degenerative disease, affects children too. Some are more at risk than others; diabetics, and the overweight and obese are particularly prone. That is worrying, as the numbers of young diabetics and the numbers of overweight and obese children – these conditions are related – are all increasing.

CRP (aka C-reactive Protein) is a marker for chronic inflammation. It is not a very good one, or the only one, but it is the most widely used at this time. A recent NHANES study, conducted in the USA in 2009, showed that heavier children have higher CRP scores, and are therefore suffering from low grade chronic inflammation. As chronic inflammation inevitably leads to progressive tissue damage, these children can expect an increased risk of chronic disease in later life.

CRP levels were higher in children with lower family income, and these differences are largely accounted for by differences in adiposity and recent illness; the children in disadvantaged familes are more likely to be overweight, to be more malnourished and to suffer from a range of illnesses.

But there is another, less obvious issue. Chronic stress, an often overlooked factor in the development of degenerative disease, places the body's inflammatory response on permanent high alert and eventually triggers chronic inflammation. This is one reason why childhood trauma leads to an average decrease in life expectancy of up to 20 years. Disadvantaged children may be more at risk of trauma but childhood trauma affects children from all social groups; and it undoubtedly affects the many immigrant children who have travelled to Europe from less stable areas of the world, and who will pose considerable health problems as they grow.

These findings are a major concern to public health workers, especially when taken into conjunction with findings from European studies that children today are less fit and less healthy than the current generation of adults were at their age. This has lead many to predict that life expectancy, which has been rising for so long, must start to fall back. We have just seen this start to happen in the USA, and the burden of lifestyle diseases will drive our public health systems to bankruptcy unless we can find a way of changing course.

Source: https://www.ncbi.nlm.nih.gov/pmc/articles/PMC2952932/

Recommended: an anti-inflammatory lifestyle and diet.

II.12 Exercise, Inflammation and Nutrition

When you exercise (and especially if you use a previously un-trained muscle group), the physical stresses placed on muscle and ligament create a certain amount of tissue damage, and this damage – together with the resulting inflammation – causes delayed onset muscle soreness (DOMS). This may not be so important for the weekend warrior, other than the fact that DOMS is one of the main reasons why people give up on exercise regimes, and cancel those New Year resolution/beer-fuelled gym memberships before the end of January. But it is critically important for athletes and sportspersons, because it damages performance. DOMS reduces running efficiency by around 3%, and at competitive levels that is the difference between between wining and losing, or between silver and gold.

A modest degree of micro-damage after exercise and moderate inflammatory responses are normal, and a good thing because they trigger a series of processes that lead to muscle repair, regeneration and improved fitness. Damaged muscle fibres are cleared away and replaced by new ones, mitochondria (the power-houses of the cell) multiply, and muscle fitness increases. This is a healthy adaptive response, and it gets better. Post-exercise pain gets less with training, as any exerciser knows, because the training process up-regulates anti-oxidant and anti-inflammatory mechanisms in the muscles, joints, ligaments and bones.

Given today's pro-inflammatory diet and lifestyles, however, post-exercise inflammation tends to be excessive. This causes excessive DOMS and can also contribute to gut and immune problems, which impair performance even further.

Restoring metabolic normality by putting the anti-inflammatory omega 3's and polyphenols back into the system is the obvious way to counter these issues, and make both training and competition more efficient and more effective.

This restorative anti-inflammatory strategy has been shown to work in top European football and basketball teams, where days lost through injury and illness have been significantly reduced, numbers of wins increased and league position improved, in some cases dramatically. Further trials are taking place in the North American ice hockey leagues, with early data showing the same results.

But is there more that can be done to enhance performance? Well, since you ask ...

To begin with, the polyphenols and omega 3's have little effect on the microbiome, which – if you eat a modern diet – is skewed towards gram-negative bacteria. These have a marked tendency to cause chronic inflammation in the gut. Conversely, certain gram-positive probiotic species have been shown to reduce inflammation, and to increase physical stamina (and mood) as a result. Anything that probiotics can do, prebiotics can do more effectively; and so a prebiotic blend is also very relevant for the serious athlete - and the keen amateur.

The next step, for those who want to take things further, would be to use an AMP-Kinase activator such as a standardised extract from the adaptogenic herb Gynostemma pentaphyllum. This is a way to enhance or mimic the positive effects of exercise, and it leads directly to enhanced muscle fitness. And for anyone who needs improved muscle bulk and strength, as well as fitness, muscle growth can be enhanced via m-TOR activation. This can be done using whole protein, or more specifically a sub-set of amino acids including leucine; and most specifically, by a metabolite of leucine called beta-hydroxy-beta-methylbutyrate (HMB).

AMP-Kinase and m-TOR are both metabolic regulators, and are both critically involved in muscle form, function and development. In the traditional sense, AMP-K is switched on by physical exercise, and makes muscle fitter. When AMP-K is activated, m-TOR is inhibited. After exercise AMP-K gradually switches off, appetite increases, foods containing protein are consumed and the resulting m-TOR activation (plus the insulin response to food) encourages muscle growth, partly by inhibiting muscle breakdown. In other words AMP-K and m-TOR are 'designed' to act cyclically, with first one and then the other being engaged to maintain, enhance and build muscle.

If you want to ride that cycle I would suggest using the AMP-K activator first, and then after 2-3 hours switching to m-TOR activation, before retiring to bed. The timing is important because the growth hormone spurt that occurs during sleep enhances the anabolic impact of m-TOR.

I first experimented with this kind of cycling back in the late '80's, and used it to transform myself from a skinny 140 lb weakling (I had been a reasonable middle distance runner) to a more muscular 195 lbs, within 5 months. It ended my running career, sadly, but it all made retrospective sense.

Middle and long distance running activates AMP-K very effectively and thus makes muscles fitter, but the constant down-regulation of M-TOR shrinks them. This is why distance runners tend to be wiry, rather than bulked up. Once I started activating M-TOR, all that changed. My muscles grew, but I was now carrying too much weight to be an effective runner.

The message, I suppose, is balance in all things. Cycle AMP-K and M-Tor to achieve the fitness level and size that works best for you, and your chosen activity. And don't over-do it.

II.13 Omega-3's and skin health

Most skin conditions have an inflammatory component. Chronic inflammation is the common element that drives reddening, swelling and itchiness of the skin. A diet with a higher omega 6:3 ratio and low levels of polyphenols increases any tendency to inflammation, and the opposite is true; a diet with a low 6:3 ratio and high levels of polyphenols acts in the opposite manner. There are various clinical trials that – while mostly badly designed in that they used only one of these nutrients (usually the omega 3's) and often used ridiculously low doses – do suggest that anti-inflammatory strategies help to reduce the inflammatory symptoms of these conditions. In my experience, a joined-up approach combining omega 3's with the right polyphenols is far more effective.

But a combined anti-inflammatory approach can do much more, because chronic inflammation is the major cause of skin ageing.

The Extra-Celluar Matrix re-visited.

Underpinning the skin, and indeed all tissues, is a 3-dimensional grid of microfibers called the extra-cellular marix. Made up of many different fiber types, it holds all our cells together and in place, correctly orientated, allowing them to communicate with each other, to function effectively and collectively, and supporting the entire micro-organisation of dermis, epidermis and deeper tissues. The extent and health of this matrix determines the skin's elasticity, its tensile strength, thickness, smoothness and ability to retain moisture. In other words, the quality of the matrix and how rapidly it degrades over time, determines skin ageing.

The matrix itself is highly dynamic, and is being constantly broken down and replaced. When the processes of breakdown and repair are in balance, the visual (and micro-structural) age of the skin does not change. But if the rates of breakdown start to accelerate, as occurs with chronic inflammation, and if the ability of the skin to make new matrix is also reduced, as occurs in malnutrition, then there is a slow erosion of the matrix over time. This leads to a gradual loss of matrix, which means that the skin thins, becomes weaker and less elastic, and loses hydration. In short, it ages, far more rapidly than it should. And because chronic inflammation and malnutrition are so common today, this is what most people experience.

This is just one more tissue where the modern lifestyle does so much damage. At one and the same time it encourages chronic inflammation (which speeds matrix breakdown), and slows the processes of tissue renewal.

Discouraging? Maybe, but from this perspective we can also see how to reverse the ageing of skin. Stop chronic inflammation with the standard combination of omega 3's and polyphenols, add all the co-factors necessary for tissue renewal, and for the final touch add topical compounds that speed matrix renewal, such as the copper peptides and the 1-3, 1-6 beta glucans.

This combination approach has been shown to reverse skin ageing dramatically – by 30% in 6 weeks.

Recommended: an anti-inflammatory lifestyle and diet. Skin care products which combine anti-inflammatory agents with matrix regenerators.

III Chapter
How to fight inflammation

"Chronic inflammation – the enemy inside you –
a slow, silent disturbance that never shuts off.
You can't feel it. You can't be tested for it.
Yet it has become a medical hot topic.
It's an underlying cause for many, many diseases."

Women's Health December 2012

"Chronic inflammation plays a central role in some of the most
challenging diseases of our time, including rheumatoid arthritis,
cancer, heart disease, diabetes, asthma, and even Alzheimer's."

Harvard Medical school statement 2018

Beating chronic inflammation via nutrition is cheap, easy, safe and considerably more effective than relying on the tender mercies of the current healthcare model. You could entrust your health to the wisdom and benevolence of our politicians and banksters, and die. Or you could take matters into your own hands, adopt an anti-inflammatory lifestyle, and live.

If that is not enough of an inducement to live a healthier lifestyle, consider two more pieces of information.

There is good evidence that our diet is not only making us sick, it is also making us stupid. Visual reaction speeds are a good measure of the functionality of the central nervous system, and correlate highly with IQ; brains that are less efficient at handling information react to stimuli more slowly. A well-controlled and rather beautiful meta-analysis of 14 age-matched studies carried out between 1884 (the earliest recorded data) and 2004 shows that our brains have indeed slowed down.

Compared to the Victorians, our visual reaction speeds have slowed by 81.4 milliseconds or 30%. This corresponds to a fall in average IQ of 14 points – a highly significant decline in our mental health, and very much in step with our declining physical health. We are eating the wrong fuel for our bodies and our brains, and creating a morass of problems that drugs and doctors cannot fix. Worryingly, the fall in IQ shows no signs of slowing down – and although every generation thinks that it is smarter than their parents, the evidence shows otherwise. Idiocracy, anyone?

If that is not enough, consider this even more existential problem. We are becoming less able to reproduce. Infertility in women is a well-known issue, but men are similarly affected. Sperm counts in the West have fallen by 60% in the last half century, and the numbers of men who are sub-fertile or infertile are increasing rapidly. If current trends continue, uncontrolled (and perhaps uncontrollable) population collapse is in our near future.

It is clear that if we wish to achieve long-term personal and public health, chronic inflammation and excess free radical action must be kept in check. There are seven steps you can take that match the main causes of inflammation. They are surprisingly easy to carry out.

ANTI-INFLAMMATORY STEP 1:
Get your diet right

You cannot stop chronological ageing. You get one year older every 365 days or so. However, given that a good deal of biological ageing is driven by chronic inflammation with a degree of free radical damage, it follows that increasing the level of anti-inflammatory and anti-oxidant nutrients in your diet will slow the rate at which you age biologically.

The key anti-inflammatory foods include fruits, vegetables and Omega 3-rich oily fish.

Fish high in Omega 3 include:

  • wild salmon (not farmed, as industrial fish feed may be high in high-Omega 6) • mackerel • herring • tuna • sardines • pilchards, oyster, crab, shrimp

Fruits with high anti-inflammatory scores include:
  • blueberries • raspberries • blackberries • strawberries • cherries • blackcurrants

High-scoring **vegetables** include:
  • broccoli • asparagus • beetroot • chard • spinach • cabbage • mushrooms (which are actually fungi, but usually live in the vegetable section)

These fruits and vegetables are all good sources of polyphenols and other phytonutrients with anti-inflammatory and anti-oxidant properties. Eating a rainbow is sound advice. Generally the more (natural) colours there are on your plate, the higher the anti-inflammatory content of your diet is.

Use Table 1 to increase anti-inflammatory foods in your diet and reduce pro-inflammatory foods. Although not a weight-loss diet in itself, many people find it easier to maintain a healthy weight on this type of food regime and most lose weight.

WILD VS FARMED FISH

Fish are no better than we are at the making Omega3 oils; fish in the wild get their Omega 3s from marine algae, which live in the Arctic waters.

Farmed fish only contain EPA and DHA if they have been fed on fish scraps which themselves contained Omega 3.

Source: "Health defence"

Can you take short chain omega 3 fatty acids from ie flax or hemp seed, which are the precursors for the longer chain omega 3's found in fish? Yes, but there is a catch. If you are consuming a lot of omega 6's, your body will not be able to use the short chain flax or hemp omega 3's UNLESS you take them in large enough amounts to dilute the 6's out. A more useful alternative for vegetarians and vegans is to take marine algal oil, which contains exactly the same omega 3's as occur in fish oil and which the body can use directly.

The Anti-Cancer Diet

The anti-cancer diet is broadly similar to the diets designed to protect against coronary artery disease, diabetes and obesity.

Table 1 Anti-inflammatory foods

	EAT MORE!	EAT LESS
Fruits	Red/black/purple fruits, all berries including strawberries, raspberries, blackberries, blueberries, elderberries, blackcurrants, citrus, plums, cherries, grapes	There are no fruits we should eat less of
Vegetables	Broccoli, chard, spinach, cabbage, collards, kale, onions, cress, carrots, sweet potatoes, garlic, peppers, mushrooms, courgettes (zucchini), celery, asparagus	Potatoes or potato products, corn or corn products, unless you are very active physically
Legumes/ Legume products	Lentils, beans, peas Tofu (from soybeans), dhal (from lentils), hummus (from chickpeas)	
Herbs and Spices	Turmeric, garlic, ginger, cayenne, chilli, curry powder, basil, thyme, black pepper, cinnamon, oregano, rosemary, nutmeg	Salt
Fats and oils	Olive oil, ghee, coconut oil. Rapeseed (canola) oil is one of the better of the common plant oils.	Other vegetable and palm oils including sunflower. Hard margarines.
Fish	Salmon (if wild), herring, tuna, mackerel, sardines, pilchards, trout, oysters, crab	Deep-fried fish, fish fingers
Meat	Game, grass-fed beef, mutton & lamb, free range chicken	Intensively farmed beef, pork or poultry. Sausages, burgers, bacon, cured meats such as hot dogs, salami
Dairy products	Real cheeses especially green & blue, unsweetened yoghurt	Sweetened yoghurt, ice cream
Breads	Wholemeal & rye in moderation, although physically active people can eat more	White (refined) flour products
Cereals	Bran cereals, low sugar muesli, porridge oats	Cornflakes, all sugared cereals
Pasta and grains	Wholemeal pasta, brown rice, quinoa	White rice, white pasta, gnocchi
Nuts and seeds	Their recorded health benefits likely relate to their polyphenol content; though they also contain omega 6 fatty acids	Salted and roasted nuts
Sweeteners	Intense sweeteners if needed. These are probably better for most than sugar or honey.	Sugar, honey, syrup, molasses
Desserts and sweets	Dark chocolate is a good source of polyphenols.	Most sweets and desserts, ice cream, baked pastries
Drinks	Water, vegetable juices, tea, coffee, milk, red wine (in moderation), fruit juices if diluted	Sugar-sweetened soft drinks, colas, spirits

EAT LESS – sugar, starchy foods, grilled and deep-fried foods, cured foods.

The ground rules for all four diets are:

- More fruits and vegetables

- More complex carbohydrates in whole grains, pulses and legumes

- Less sugar and salt

- Less smoked and/or pickled foods

- Less foods cooked at high temperature ie barbecued and fried foods

There should be plenty of fruits, nuts, grains, legumes and vegetables on the menu, as all of these contain many different anti-cancer compounds. Fruits are excellent sources of protective phytonutrients such as the carotenoids, xanthophylls and polyphenols, as well as several vitamins and minerals. Grains and nuts are good sources of Vitamin E and polyphenols, including unique anti-inflammatory agents such as the avenanthramides, found in oats.

Vegetables, and spices such as rosemary and turmeric provide not only anti-inflammatory polyphenols, but also compounds which boost the Phase 2 enzymes needed in the body to detoxify toxins and carcinogens; as do the brassica and cruciderous vegetables. Both fruits and vegetables provide polyphenols and carotenoids, while peas and beans are good sources of lectins (protease inhibitors which work together with the polyphenols to inhibit the tissue-damaging MMP enzymes). Plant foods also provide prebiotic dietary fibres, which reduce chronic inflammation in the large bowel and have anti-cancer effects of their own. Finally, they are a good source of B vitamins folic acid and niacin important because folate and/or niacin depletion increases the risk of DNA damage.

Some cooking tips

• Use fewer Omega 6 polyunsaturated plant oils; switch to (mono-unsaturated) olive oil or saturated fats.

• Reduce foods cooked at high temperatures (grilled, fried, barbe-cued, roasted). Instead, stew, slow-cook, stir-fry or sauté quickly.

• Steam or microwave vegetables.

• Rub joints for roasting with thyme and/or oregano, herbs that help counteract the formation of AGE products. Do not use honey to coat or glaze meat as this encourages AGEs.

Omega 3's, Polyphenols – or Both

As chronic inflammation has two phases (the first being influenced by the 6:3 ratio and the 2nd by polyphenols), it makes sense to take both omega 3's AND polyphenols. It makes even more sense to take them together. Lipid-soluble polyphenols such as those from olives act as chaperones to the omega 3's, protecting them and keeping them intact until they can get to all the body's cells where they switch off the upper half of the inflammazone. Once the polyphenols have arrived at the cell, they have another function; they switch off the lower half of the inflammazone.

If you take enough polyphenols, they can do the job all by themselves. I have seen this in India, for example, where there are no cold ocean waters and hence no oily fish. This is why South-East Asians have such high omega 6:3 ratios – 100:1 is not uncommon. The traditional Indian diet, however, contains huge amounts of spices which contain very high levels of polyphenols. Anyone who has cooked Indian dishes will know that where the Western chef uses a pinch or two of spice, Indian chefs use them by the tablespoon. This is why, despite very high omega 6:3 ratios, it is perfectly possible for Indians to avoid inflammageing.

But there is a catch. Unlike the omega 3's, most polyphenols are not stored in the body. That means they must be consumed very regularly, because when you stop eating them they quickly disappear from the tissues. When the junk food franchises came to India and the urban young abandoned their traditional eating habits, degenerative diseases multiplied, occurring at ever-younger ages and overwhelming their health care systems.

In North America and Europe, many people consume at least some omega 3's from seafoods. Omega 3's are built into the cell membrane of our cells, and can remain there for long periods of time. This means that we are not so dependent on frequent 'doses' of polyphenols, and are slightly less vulnerable to junk food. But there is no doubt that it harms us as well.

ANTI-INFLAMMATORY STEP 2:
Take an anti-inflammatory supplement

Conventional daily A-Z vitamin and mineral tablets provide a baseline of those micronutrients for which there are Recommended Daily Amounts (RDAs), but will do little or nothing to reduce chronic inflammation.

This is one reason why studies on simple vitamin and mineral supplements show no reduction in age-related disease.

Another reason is that there are many essential and conditionally essential micronutrients that we need to stay healthy, but which do not have RDA's yet. For example, we need cyanogens, caro-tenoids (and not just beta carotene), xanthophylls, polyphenols, methyl group donors, at least 4 fiber types – the list goes on and on.

Old school nutritionists and uninformed doctors still parrot the line that you can get all you need from a well-balanced diet, but while this was undoubtedly true in earlier ages, it is no longer helpful or accurate. You can get everything you need from a carefully balanced diet,

IF you are consuming 3500 calories a day or more, and living on a diet rich in fruit, vegetables, yeast, chicken livers and oily fish.

But in today's age of processed and ultra-processed foods, this is not what most people eat. Moreover, very few are consuming 3500 calories / day, as with today's low energy lifestyle, this would be a fast route to overweight and obesity.

In a sedentary population with low energy requirements, and where 2000 to 2500 calories per day is considered normal, it is no longer possible to get everything needed for long-term health from even a well-balanced diet.

The 'well-balanced diet' will generally prevent outright deficiency, but it will not prevent micro- and phyto-nutrient depletion, and thus cannot protect against chronic inflammation, or degenerative disease.

The simple truth is that we eat too many foods with a low nutrient density, and we do not eat enough of them, to obtain all we need from our diet. Supplements have become critically important. But to have any effect, these must contain far more than a mere list of vitamins and minerals. They must provide a comprehensive micro- and phyto-nutrient support program.

This will not fit into a single tablet, unless it is the size of a golf ball – so it has to be divided into a larger number of tablets. Ideally, they should be consumed at different times during the day, with meals, to ensure optimal uptake and utilisation within the body. And even this will not be enough unless they are combined with fish oils and dietary fibers. The right (effective) doses of these cannot be stuffed into a capsule or tablet, and require different delivery systems in liquid, powder or food format.

What will such comprehensive micro- and phyto-nutrient support do for your health? It's hard to answer this question, but in my own researches into Victorian public health, this level of nutrition was linked to a near 90% reduction in lifestyle disease. It was also associated with an almost complete absence of immunological problems.

Skeptics will point out that there was more to the Victorian lifestyle than their diet, and I would agree. They were also very active, they did not use much tobacco or alcohol, and they did not use high temperature cooking techniques. But there is another line of evidence, from pre-clinical studies carried out at McMaster University (and referred to above). The scientists there found that this kind of nutrition extended life in mice by up to 28% (another 20 years in human terms), enabled faster learning, and stopped all the signs of brain ageing.

So the the standard A-Z, which is little more than a nutritional foundation, I would add ...

1. A ground floor consisting of an extensive range of phytonutrients. This should include lycopene, alpha as well as beta carotene, lutein, zeaxanthin, all 8 forms of vitamin E and both water- and fat-soluble polyphenols.

2. A first floor designed to support innate immune function. This is essential because when inflammation is excessively damped, this can theoretically lead to impaired immune function.

The innate immune system is far more important for our heath than the adaptive immune system, and can be divided into two forms of defences – cellular and humoral. The appropriate nutrients here are the 1-3, 1-6 beta glucans (derived from bakers yeast), and a cyanogen such as broccoli or apple seed extract, which respectively support cellular and humoral elements of the innate immune system. More information on these (and on all the other essential nutrients) can be found below, and on the international database PubMed.

ANTI-INFLAMMATORY STEP 3:
A little more exercise, please!

Moderate exercise increases your health prospects, in part because it has anti-inflammatory effects. The standard advice is to take 30 minutes of exercise, five times a week, at a level that raises your heart rate.

People who exercise at around this level have lower rates of heart disease, cancer, diabetes and dementia.

However, you can over-dose. Intense exercise can trigger inflammation and excessive free radicals, so take anti-inflammatory supplements to counter negative effects.

ANTI-INFLAMMATORY STEP 4:
Lose weight if you need to

If you carry excess weight, slim down in a gradual and sustainable way. There is evidence that yo-yo dieting is intrinsically pro-inflammatory, so avoid crash diets.

Support any weight-loss regime with a supplement that includes a full range of anti-inflammatory nutrients and phyto-nutrients, as these all tend to be low in calorie-restricted diets.

ANTI-INFLAMMATORY STEP 5:
Give your innate immune system the best chance of clearing any infection.

If a harmful microorganism invades the body and the acute inflammatory response is insufficient to clear that threat, the infectious agent may linger on. The body will then switch over to a chronic inflammatory response that will increase the risk of progressive tissue damage leading to degenerative diseases. This is why, for example, poor oral hygiene and subsequent chronic gingival (gum) inflammation are linked to heart disease.

It is therefore important to ensure that your acute immune response is efficient in fully clearing infections. The most effective and natural way to boost your immunity is to take 1-3, 1-6 beta glucans. These are polysaccharides, derived from bakers' yeast, that have been proven to increase the effectiveness of your front-line immune system defence against bacteria and viruses.

The 1-3, 1-6 beta glucans (not to be confused with the 1-3, 1-4 beta glucans in oats and other cereals) have been tested, in animal models, against a wide range of pathogens from E.coli to flu viruses and even the deadly anthrax bacillus, and shown to be highly protective against all of them. When the Canadian Department of Defence was searching for an immune enhancer that could help counteract radiation, they tested over 100 products. 1-3, 1-6 beta glucans derived from bakers' yeast came out on top. In my view the beta glucans are best combined with a cyanogen, which is needed by the immunoprotective enzyme lactoperoxidase.

A comprehensive anti-inflammatory supplement will help to protect against long-term chronic inflammation. A 1-3, 1-6 beta glucan / cyanogen supplement is designed to enhance the immune system's short-term acute response. The combination has exciting potential in reducing our overall burden of degenerative, infectious and allergic disease.

ANTI-INFLAMMATORY STEP 6.

Stop smoking, but you already knew that. Minimise exposure to air pollution where possible.

ANTI-INFLAMMATORY STEP 7.

De-stress, if you need to. Chronic stress contributes to the development of degenerative disease, because it places the body's inflammatory response on permanent high alert. Meditate, paint, garden, live mindfully. For a short-cut, try saffron. Standardised extracts of saffron have been shown to reduce anxiety, low mood and deoression, improve sleep and reduce stress.

Last Word:

A lifestyle approach combining a healthy diet, regular movement and stress reduction improves quality of life, reduces chronic inflammation and all-cause mortality. It will improve both health and life expectancy.

That's a lot to take on faith. This booklet attempts to provide an accessible working summary of current research, and practical suggestions for improving your health. It's a lot of ground to cover, so while the text is wide it is also shallow. For those who want more than a general introduction, and are interested in the details of the research, the parent book 'Out of the Fire' (also by Paul Clayton) provides this, together with an extensive list of the original references from which this work derives.

'If you found this book interesting but would like to see the evidence, take a look at Paul Clayton's companion book, Out of the Fire. This is a much more detailed review of chronic inflammation, with an extensive bibliography.'

Glossary

1-3, 1-4 beta glucan. A carbohydrate, this indigestible fiber occurs in cereals such as oats. It is not broken down to glucose, and is thus suitable for diabetics. It acts as a prebiotic, supporting the growth of healthy bacteria in the gut.

1-3, 1-6 beta glucan. A related carbohydrate, this indigestible fiber occurs in the cell walls of yeast. It is a highly effective immune-modulator, and raises resistance to infection. It also has powerful anti-allergy effects.

AA. Arachidonic acid. A highly unsaturated (and essential) Omega 6 fatty acid, occurring in meat and dairy products. It is also formed in the body from the shorter chain LA (Linoleic Acid) found in plant oils. It is essential for cell growth and function, but when present in excess, as it inevitably is in modern diets, it has marked pro-inflammatory effects.

AGE. Advanced Glycation End Products are formed when foods containing sugars and starches are heated. AGE compounds are highly pro-inflammatory.

ALA. Alpha Linolenic Acid is an omega 3 fatty acid found in many plant foods, and can be metabolized in the body to form the essential Omega 3 fatty acids EPA and DHA. It is not a good source of these however, as our ability to transform ALA into DHA and EPA is very limited.

ALE. Advanced Lipoxidation End Products are formed when foods containing oils and fats are over-heated. ALE compounds are highly pro-inflammatory.

Angiogenesis. Angiogenesis is the process of new blood vessel formation. This is essential for the normal growth of tissues, but it is also vital for the growth of tumours.

Carotene. Alpha- and beta-carotene are coloured compounds found in many fruits and vegetables. Both carotenes have multiple functions in the body, including anti-inflammatory and cancer-fighting properties.

CRP. C-Reactive Protein is formed in the liver as a response to inflammation occurring anywhere in the body. It is used by doctors to monitor inflammation, but neither CRP nor hsCRP is insufficiently sensitive to diagnose the low, sustained levels of chronic inflammation that drive degenerative diseases.

Cyanogen. Cyanogens are compounds in the diet which, when ingested, release small amounts of thiocyanates. Thiocyanates are essential substrates for the enxyme lactoperoxidase, which defends us against bacterial and viral invaders.

DHA. Docahexaenoic Acid, one of the two essential omega 3 fatty acids. Found in seafoods, and especially oily fish, this compound has powerful anti-inflammatory effects and is essential for the growth and health of tissues.

Extra-Cellular Matrix (ECM). A fine, three-dimensional mesh of microfibers which permeates all tissue and organs, providing a 'soft skeleton' which gives them structure and allows them to function. The fibers include a range of collagens, glycosaminoglycans and proteoglycans, elastin and hyaluronic acid. The propertions of these fibers differs in different tissues.

EPA. Eicosapentaenoic Acid, the second of the two essential omega 3 fatty acids. Found in seafoods, and especially oily fish, this compound has powerful anti-inflammatory effects and is also essential for the growth and health of tissues.

HUFA. Highly Unsaturated Fatty Acids. These include the Omega 3 fatty acids DHA and EPA, and the Omega 6 fatty acid AA.

Inflammazone. This is shorthand used to describe some of the intra-cellular machinery that drives chronic inflammation. It can be functionally divided into two compartments, an upper and a lower, which are modified by the Omega 6:3 ratio and by polyphenols respectively. A diet designed to reduce chronic inflammation effectively should modify activity in both compartments.

Insulin resistance - in this situation the muscles do not respond to insulin, leading to increased levels of glucose in the blood and increased inflammatory stress. This metabolic imbalance, if allowed to continue for long periods of time, increases the risk of many degenerative conditions.

Junk foods. A difficult term to define, but broadly these are foods which contain excessive amounts empty calories (ie sugars, starches and plant oils), an unhealthy balance of electrolyes (ie too much salt), few if any anti-inflammatory compounds and high levels of pro-inflammatory compounds such as ALA, AGE's and ALE's. Fries and burgers are good examples of junk foods.

LA. Linoleic Acid, a short chain Omega 6 fatty acid found in plant oils.

Lactoperoxidase. This enzyme is part of the innate immune system, and an important defence against infection in the eyes, ears, nose, throat, lungs, gut, urinary tract and mammary glands.

Lectin. Lectins are a wide range of proteins mostly from plant foods that bind to carbohydrates and specifically to sugar molecules in the body. By doing so, they exert multiple effects. While some lectins are highly poisonous (such as ricin, from the castor oil plant), others have beneficial effects. Lectins from peas and beans, for example, prevent the activation of the tissue-destructive MMP enzymes.

Lycopene. A red compound found in tomatoes and watermelon, this phytonutrient has anti-inflammatory and anti-cancer properties.

Lutein. A yellowish compound found in foods such as kale, corn and avocado, lutein is essential for eye health. It also has anti-inflammatory and anti-cancer properties.

Malnutrition Type A - typically combines a deficiency of a vitamin such as vitamin C, or a trace element such as iodine, with calorie deficit and therefore weight loss. Most often seen in developing countries.

Malnutrition Type B - usually combines sub-optimal levels of many micronutrients including vitamins, trace elements, omega 3 fatty acids, prebiotic fibers, and many phytonutrients, with calorie excess, and therefore weight gain. Commonly found in developed nations.

Monounsaturated fatty acid. These are fatty acids with only one double bond, which makes them fairly resistant to oxidation. Oleic acid (in olive oil and other sources) is a good example, and is thought to exert beneficial effects on blood chemistry.

Matrix Metallo-Proteases (MMP's). MMP enzymes play a critically important role in the growth and development of tissues, but when released in excessive amounts (as in chronic inflammation) they lead to the slow erosion of tissue. This is what drives the progressive loss of function and the emergence of symptoms that characterize the degenerative diseases. They are inhibited by polyphenols.

Polyphenol. A huge family of compounds found in plant foods, these compounds have multiple effects in the body, which are predominantly protective. They include the inhibition of inflammation, and many anti-cancer effects. Most are water-soluble, and a valuable few are fat-soluble; we need both for the best chance of good health. Best sources of the fat-soluble polyphenols include pre-harvest olive oil and some cold-water seaweeds. Good sources of the water-soluble polyphenols include tea, coffee, cocoa and spices such as turmeric, thyme and marjoram.

Polyunsaturated fatty acid. Fatty acids that contain several double bonds, which make them prone to oxidation. PUFA's can be either Omega 6 or Omega 3.

Preclinical. Early stage in the progression of a disease, which is not yet advanced enough to cause symptoms. This phase may last for decades, and occurs in those whose lifestyles promote chronic inflammation.

Zeaxanthin. A yellow compound found in foods such as kale, corn and wolfberries, zeaxanthin is essential for eye health. It also has anti-inflammatory and anti-cancer properties.

References

Akbaraly T, Sabia S, Hagger-Johnson G, Tabak AG, Shipley MJ, Jokela M, Brunner EJ, Hamer M, Batty GD, Singh-Manoux A, Kivimaki M. Does overall diet in midlife predict future aging phenotypes? A cohort study. Am J Med. 2013 May;126(5):411-419.

Bahadoran Z, Mirmiran P, Azizi F. Fast Food Pattern and Cardiometabolic Disorders: A Review of Current Studies. Health Promot Perspect. 2016 Jan 30;5(4):231-40.

Benros ME, Waltoft BL, Nordentoft M, Ostergaard SD, Eaton WW, Krogh J, Mortensen PB. Autoimmune diseases and severe infections as risk factors for mood disorders: a nationwide study. JAMA Psychiatry. 2013 Aug;70(8):812-20.

Clayton PR, Ladi S. From alga to omega; have we reached peak (fish) oil? Journal of the Royal Society of Medicine; 2015, Vol. 108(9) 351–357

Clayton P, Rowbotham J. An unsuitable and degraded diet? Part one: public health lessons from the mid-Victorian working class diet. J R Soc Med. 2008 Jun;101(6):282-9.

Clayton P, Rowbotham J. An unsuitable and degraded diet? Part two: realities of the mid-Victorian diet. J R Soc Med. 2008 Jul;101(7):350-7.

Clayton P, Rowbotham J. How the mid-Victorians worked, ate and died. Int J Environ Res Public Health. 2009 Mar; 6(3):1235-53.

Dowd JB, Zajacova A, Aiello AE. Predictors of Inlammation in U.S. Children Aged 3–16 Years: Am J Prev Med. 2010 Oct; 39(4): 314–320.

Jelodar G, Javid Z, Sahraian A, Jelodar S. Saffron improved depression and reduced homocysteine level in patients with major depression: A Randomized, double-blind study. Avicenna J Phytomed. 2018 Jan-Feb;8(1):43-50.

Mediterranean Diet, Lifestyle Factors, and 10-Year Mortality in Elderly European Men and Women; The HALE Project. Knoops K, de Groot L, Kromhout D, Perrin A-E, Moreiras-Varela O, Menotti A, van Staveren WA et al. JAMA. 2004;292(12):1433-1439.

Laurin D, David Curb J, Masaki KH, White LR, Launer LJ. Midlife C-reactive protein and risk of cognitive decline: a 31-year follow-up. Neurobiol Aging. 2009 Nov;30(11):1724-7.

Lemon JA, Aksenov V, Samigullina R, Aksenov S, Rodgers WH, Rollo CD, Boreham DR. A multi-ingredient dietary supplement abolishes large-scale brain cell loss, improves sensory function, and prevents neuronal atrophy in aging mice. Environ Mol Mutagen. 2016 Jun; 57(5):382-404.

Levine H, Jørgensen N, Martino-Andrade A, Mendiola J, Weksler-Derri D et al. Temporal trends in sperm count: a systematic review and meta-regression analysis. *Human Reproduction Update* 23(6), 646–659.

Lopresti AL, Drummond PD. Efficacy of curcumin, and a saffron/curcumin combination for the treatment of major depression: A randomised, double-blind, placebo-controlled study. J Affect Disord. 2017 Jan 1;207:188-196.

Mancini SJ, White AD, Bijland S, Rutherford C, Graham D, Richter EA, Viollet B, Touyz RM, Palmer TM, Salt IP. Activation of AMP-activated protein kinase rapidly suppresses multiple pro-inflammatory pathways in adipocytes including IL-1 receptor-associated kinase-4 phosphorylation. Mol Cell Endocrinol. 2017 Jan 15;440:44-56.

Michelson PH, Williams LW, Benjamin DK, Barnato AE. Obesity, inflammation, and asthma severity in childhood: data from the National Health and Nutrition Examination Survey 2001-2004. Ann Allergy Asthma Immunol. 2009 Nov;103(5):381-5.

Monteiro CA, Moubarac J-C, Bertazz R. Household availability of ultra-processed foods and obesity in nineteen European countries. Public Health Nutrition ß21 (1) (Ultra Processed Foods) Jan 2018 , pp. 18-26

Out of the Fire. Clayton P, PharmacoNutrition Press HK, 2016

Oyebode OC, Gordon-Dseagu V, Walker A, Mindell JS. Fruit and vegetable consumption and all-cause, cancer and CVD mortality: analysis of Health Survey for England data. J Epidemiol Community Health. 2014 Sep;68(9):856-62.

Rojas A, Añazco C, González I, Paulina A. Extracellular matrix glycation and RAGE activation. A missing piece in the puzzle of the association between diabetes and cancer. Carcinogenesis. 2018, bgy012, https://doi.org/10.1093/carcin/bgy012

Rowbotham J, Clayton P. An unsuitable and degraded diet? Part three: Victorian consumption patterns and their health benefits. J R Soc Med. 2008 Sep;101(9):454-62.

Schacter E, Weitzman SA. Chronic Inflammatio and Cancer. Cacer Network 2001
http://www.cancernetwork.com/review-article/chronic-inflammation-and-cancer

Shivappa N, Hebert JR, Kivimaki M, Akbaraly T. Alternate Healthy Eating Index 2010, Dietary Inflammatory Index and risk of mortality: results from the Whitehall II cohort study and meta-analysis of previous Dietary Inflammatory Index and mortality studies. Br J Nutr. 2017 Aug;118(3):210-221

Steele EM, Baraldi LG, da Costa Louzada ML, Moubarac J-C, Mozaffarian D, Augusto Monteiro C. Ultra-processed foods and added sugars in the US diet: evidence from a nationally representative cross-sectional study BMJ Open. 2016; 6(3): e009892

Tomkinson GR, Lang JJ, Tremblay MS. Temporal trends in the cardiorespiratory fitness of children and adolescents representing 19 high-income and upper middle-income countries between 1981 and 2014. Br J Sports Med. 2017 Oct 30. pii: bjsports-2017-097982.

Woodley of Menie MA, te Nijenhuis J, Murphy R. The Victorians were still faster than us. Commentary: Factors influencing the latency of simple reaction time. Front Hum Neurosci. 2015; 9: 452. 88

Notes